ASK THE EXPERTS

Expert Answers about Your Diabetes

FROM THE PAGES OF

Diabetes
FORECAST

American
Diabetes
Association

Director, Book Publishing, Abe Ogden; *Managing Editor,* Greg Guthrie; *Acquisitions Editor,* Victor Van Beuren; *Editor,* Lauren Wilson; *Production Manager,* Melissa Sprott; *Composition,* American Diabetes Association; *Cover Design,* Sport Creative; *Printer,* Versa Press, Inc.

Printed in the United States of America
1 3 5 7 9 10 8 6 4 2

The suggestions and information contained in this publication are generally consistent with the *Clinical Practice Recommendations* and other policies of the American Diabetes Association, but they do not represent the policy or position of the Association or any of its boards or committees. Reasonable steps have been taken to ensure the accuracy of the information presented. However, the American Diabetes Association cannot ensure the safety or efficacy of any product or service described in this publication. Individuals are advised to consult a physician or other appropriate health care professional before undertaking any diet or exercise program or taking any medication referred to in this publication. Professionals must use and apply their own professional judgment, experience, and training and should not rely solely on the information contained in this publication before prescribing any diet, exercise, or medication. The American Diabetes Association—its officers, directors, employees, volunteers, and members—assumes no responsibility or liability for personal or other injury, loss, or damage that may result from the suggestions or information in this publication.

⊗ The paper in this publication meets the requirements of the ANSI Standard Z39.48-1992 (permanence of paper).

ADA titles may be purchased for business or promotional use or for special sales. To purchase more than 50 copies of this book at a discount, or for custom editions of this book with your logo, contact the American Diabetes Association at the address below, at booksales@diabetes.org, or by calling 703-299-2046.

American Diabetes Association
1701 North Beauregard Street
Alexandria, Virginia 22311

DOI: 10.2337/9781580405393

Library of Congress Cataloging-in-Publication Data

Ask the experts : expert answers about your diabetes from the pages of Diabetes forecast.
    pages cm
 Summary: "This book is a compilation of questions sent in to the editors of Diabetes Forecast. They were from diabetes patients and were chosen to provide information on general issues that diabetics face"-- Provided by publisher.
  ISBN 978-1-58040-539-3 (pbk.)
  1. Diabetes--Miscellanea. I. American Diabetes Association. II. Diabetes forecast.
  RC660.A685 2014
  616.4'62--dc23
                    2013046542

CONTENTS

CONTRIBUTORS

Nicholas Argento, MD
Diabetes Technology Director
Maryland Endocrine and Diabetes
Columbia, MD
Diabetes Advisor
Howard County General Hospital
Columbia, MD

Mary M. Austin, RD, MA, CDE, FAADE
President, The Austin Group, LLC
Shelby Township, MI

Roger P. Austin, MS, RPh, CDE
Clinical Pharmacy Specialist—Diabetes
Henry Ford Health System
Sterling Heights, MI

David E. Bruns, MD
Professor of Pathology
Director of Clinical Chemistry
Associate Director of Molecular Diagnostics
Department of Pathology
University of Virginia School of Medicine and Health System
Charlottesville, VA

Belinda Childs, APRN, MN, BC-ADM, CDE
Diabetes Clinical Nurse Specialist
Director, Clinical and Research Services
MidAmerica Diabetes Associates, PA
Wichita, KS

Paul Ciechanowski, MD, MPH

Associate Professor
Psychiatry and Behavioral Sciences
Director, UW Training Xchange,
    Center for Commercialization
Team Psychiatrist, Diabetes Care Center,
    UW Medical Center
University of Washington
Seattle, WA

Mary de Groot, PhD

Associate Professor of Medicine
Division of Endocrinology and Metabolism
Associate Director
Diabetes Translational Research Center
Indiana University
Indianapolis, IN

Alison B. Evert, MS, RD, CDE

Diabetes Nutrition Educator
Coordinator of Diabetes Education Programs
Diabetes Care Center
University of Washington Medical Center
Seattle, WA

Robert A. Gabbay, MD, PhD

Chief Medical Officer
Senior Vice President
Joslin Diabetes Center
Harvard Medical School
Boston, MA

Bret Goodpaster, PhD

Professor
Senior Investigator
Translational Research Institute
    for Metabolism and Diabetes
Florida Hospital and Sanford-Burnham Medical
    Research Institute
Orlando, FL

Katie Hathaway, JD

Managing Director, Legal Advocacy
American Diabetes Association
Alexandria, VA

M. Sue Kirkman, MD
Professor of Medicine
Division of Endocrinology and Metabolism
University of North Carolina School of Medicine
Chapel Hill, NC

Janis McWilliams, RN, MSN, CDE, BC-ADM
Consultant
Pittsburgh, PA

Meghann Moore, RD, CDE, MPH
Nutrition Management Consultant
Coordinator, Diabetes Self-Management Education Program
The Polyclinic
Seattle, WA

Christy Parkin, MSN, RN, CDE
Health Management Resources, Inc.
Diabetes Education and Consulting Services
Indianapolis, IN

Paris Roach, MD
Associate Professor of Clinical Medicine
Fellowship Program Director
Department of Medicine
Division of Endocrinology and Metabolism
Indiana University School of Medicine
Indianapolis, IN

Henry Rodriguez, MD
Professor of Pediatrics
Clinical Director, USF Diabetes Center
University of South Florida College of Medicine
Tampa, FL

Janis Roszler, MSFT, RD, LD/N, CDE, FAND
2008–2009 Diabetes Educator of the Year
    (American Association of Diabetes Educators)
Marriage and Family Therapist
Miami/Fort Lauderdale, FL

Lee J. Sanders, DPM
Consultant, VA Medical Center
Lebanon, PA
Clinical Professor (Adjunct)
Department of Podiatric Medicine
Temple University School of Podiatric Medicine
Philadelphia, PA

David A. Simmons, MD
VP, Head, Global Medical and Clinical Affairs
Bayer Diabetes Care
Whippany, NJ

Cassandra L. Verdi, MPH, RD
Associate Director of Nutrition and Medical Affairs
American Diabetes Association
Alexandria, VA

Nina Watson, MSN, RN, CDE, Retired Lt. Col., USAF
Diabetes Center of Excellence
Wilford Hall Ambulatory Surgical Center
Lackland Air Force Base, TX

Jill Weisenberger, MS, RDN, CDE
Registered Dietitian Nutritionist
Author of *Diabetes Weight Loss—Week by Week*
Newport News, VA

Madelyn L. Wheeler, MS, RDN, CD, FADA, FAND
Co-Owner
Nutritional Computing Concepts
Zionsville, IN

Craig Williams, PharmD
Clinical Professor of Pharmacy
Oregon State University/Oregon Health & Science University
    College of Pharmacy
Clinical Associate Professor of Medicine
Oregon Health & Science University School of Medicine
Portland, OR

General Diabetes Questions

1

Can Diabetes Symptoms Develop Suddenly?

I haven't experienced any symptoms of diabetes in the past, but just in the last week or so, I have seen a dramatic increase in my urination frequency: I have to go about once an hour. And I seem to be constantly thirsty. Is it possible that symptoms of diabetes could materialize virtually overnight?

Name Withheld

Janis McWilliams, RN, MSN, CDE, BC-ADM, responds: Yes, in type 1 diabetes in particular, the onset of symptoms like frequent urination and extreme thirst can be very sudden. In type 2 diabetes, the symptoms tend to come about more gradually, and sometimes there are no signs at all. People who have symptoms should contact their health-care provider immediately for an accurate diagnosis. Keep in mind that these symptoms could signal other problems too.

In type 1 diabetes, other symptoms to watch for include unexplained weight loss, lethargy, drowsiness, and hunger. Symptoms sometimes occur after a viral illness. In some cases, a person may reach the point of diabetic ketoacidosis (DKA) before a type 1 diagnosis is made. DKA occurs when blood glucose is dangerously high and the body can't get nutrients into the cells because of the absence of insulin. The body then breaks down muscle and fat for energy, causing an accumulation of dangerous waste products called ketones in the blood and urine. Symptoms of DKA include a fruity odor on the breath; heavy, strained breathing; and vomiting. If left untreated, DKA can result in a dazed state, unconsciousness, and even death.

Type 2 diabetes usually has a slower onset and can often go undiagnosed. But many people do have symptoms like extreme thirst and frequent urination. Other signs include sores that won't heal, frequent infections (including vaginal infections in some women), and changes in vision. Some patients actually go to the doctor with symptoms resulting from the complications of diabetes, like tingling in the feet (neuropathy) or vision loss (retinopathy), without knowing they have the disease. This is why screening people who are at risk for diabetes is so important. The best way to avoid complications is to get blood glucose under control before symptoms arise.

A final note about type 1 diabetes: some people have a "honeymoon" period, a brief remission of symptoms while the pancreas is still secreting some insulin. The honeymoon phase typically occurs after insulin treatment has been started. A honeymoon can last as little as a week or even up to a year. But the absence of symptoms doesn't mean the diabetes is gone. The pancreas will eventually be unable to secrete insulin, and, if untreated, the symptoms will return.

Can Stress and Depression Cause Type 2 Diabetes?

Can stress trigger the onset of type 2 diabetes in someone who is not obese? I have been active most of my life, but slowed down in my desk job over the past few years. I was diagnosed with type 2 diabetes in 2006, and the only link that seems plausible to me is that at that time I was suffering from deep depression, which was later diagnosed as post-traumatic stress disorder.

Name Withheld

Mary de Groot, PhD, responds: Over the past 20 years, we have learned that people with diabetes are twice as likely to experience depression as people without diabetes. When people with diabetes have depression, it is more difficult to manage blood glucose and to stick to treatment plans like medication and regular exercise. Studies have shown depression to be associated with diabetes complications and even early death. Most recently, a series of studies in which individuals were followed over a period of 10–20 years found that people who have a history of major depression have an increased risk of developing type 2 diabetes later in life.

We do not yet know definitively how depression, stress, and diabetes are related. But here's the good news: depression can be successfully treated in people with diabetes. There are a number of antidepressant medications that have been found to be effective. It is important to talk with your doctor about these medications and which one or ones may be the best for you. It is also important to keep in mind that antidepressant medications need time to take effect (typically 2–6 weeks), should be taken as prescribed (daily), and should be changed or stopped only on the advice of your health-care provider. It is not uncommon for patients to be prescribed more than one medication before finding the right fit to treat their depression.

Another effective form of treatment for depression in people with type 2 diabetes is "talk therapy," or cognitive behavioral therapy. Studies have shown that people who meet with a therapist weekly for 8–16 weeks learn to manage depressive symptoms more effectively by using tools that address common thoughts, feelings, and behaviors that come with depression. Exercise has also been found to be an effective treatment when combined with talk therapy.

It is important to tell your health-care provider about changes in your mood so that you may talk together about the treatment options that are best suited for you. With help from your provider, it is possible to feel better with diabetes.

Does My Age of Diagnosis Affect My Children's Risk?

I s there any correlation between being diagnosed with type 1 diabetes at a later age and less risk that your children will develop diabetes? I was diagnosed at 31.

R. D., Woodridge, IL

Janis McWilliams, RN, MSN, CDE, BC-ADM, responds: Yes, there is evidence that a later age of diagnosis reduces your children's risk of developing type 1 diabetes.

What to Know: Genes alone aren't enough to cause diabetes. People inherit a predisposition to develop type 1 diabetes, and then something in their environment must trigger the disease. Scientists are trying to discover what the triggers are; the suspects include viruses.

Fathers with type 1 diabetes have a greater chance than mothers of having a child who develops the disease. Although the evidence on exact risk rates is not yet crystal clear, the best data show that, in general, the odds of a man with type 1 diabetes having a child with type 1 diabetes are 1 in 17, according to the American Diabetes Association. If you are a woman with type 1 diabetes and your child was born before you were 25 years old, your child's risk is estimated at 1 in 25; if your child was born after you turned 25 years old, your child's risk is believed to be 1 in 100.

A child's risk for developing type 1 is less if the parent developed diabetes at an older age. A child's risk is doubled, the Association says, if the parent developed type 1 diabetes before age 11. If both parents have type 1 diabetes, the risk to the child is estimated at 10–25%.

Find Out More: Most people who develop type 1 diabetes have immune markers in their blood, such as certain antibodies and enzymes. Blood tests for such markers or for specific genes can gauge the risk for developing type 1 diabetes in relatives of people with the disease.

Takeaways: Relatives of people with type 1 diabetes may be able to participate in studies (and assess their own risk) through TrialNet, a network of researchers dedicated to the study, prevention, and early treatment of type 1 diabetes. For details, go to www.diabetestrialnet.org.

How Can I Find an Endocrinologist?

How do you find an endocrinologist when you need an answer to a diabetes problem that other doctors cannot provide? My internist recently sent a referral to yet another endocrinologist and, after a month, there has been no response.

When I have tried to find an endocrinologist before, the first thing I am asked is whether I am on Medicare. My reply in the affirmative has always been my last contact with that endocrinologist. What can I do?

B. H., Boise, ID

R. Mack Harrell, MD, FACP, FACE, responds:

What to Know: Our best guess is that there are approximately 5,000 practicing endocrinologists in the United States and about 26 million people with diabetes and 79 million with prediabetes. This effectively means that there is one endocrinologist for every 5,200 people with diabetes. As you can imagine, this demand for diabetes services far exceeds what any single endocrinologist can provide, because the average physician can usually handle no more than 500–750 people with this disease in his or her practice.

Diabetes care is not easy. The Medicare system requires paperwork up to four times yearly explaining the patient's use of blood glucose supplies, and expensive medications require physician letters of medical necessity whenever they are renewed. Most patients are seen in the office at least four times a year, and many endocrinologists ask their patients to fax in blood glucose numbers every 2–4 weeks to make sure that glucose control is stable. All of this makes diabetes care extremely time consuming and expensive for a physician and his or her office.

Possible Solutions: All that said, you should still be able to find an endocrinologist in your area who can help you. If you are not online yourself, just have an Internet-savvy friend or relative help you go on the Internet and visit the American Association of Clinical Endocrinologists website. Look for the "Find an Endocrinologist" button on the right side of the home page. You can search for an endocrinologist in your area by location, area of interest, or both. You may also want to consider consulting a nurse practitioner or certified diabetes educator. They may be able to help you with your diabetes questions until you find an endocrinologist.

Can Diabetes Affect My Mood?

I was recently diagnosed with type 2 diabetes. I am on two different types of insulin, NovoLog and Levemir (insulin detemir). Can diabetes have a bearing on mood or cause sudden "bad mood episodes"?

Name Withheld

Mary de Groot, PhD, responds: Mood changes are a common experience in people with either type 1 or type 2 diabetes. Changes in mood can be attributed to various factors, including rapid changes in blood glucose, the stresses and strains of managing diabetes every day, or depression.

What to Know: Some people experience increased irritable or sad moods when they have a rapid change in their blood glucose level. This can be either a decrease from their usual level that is still in the normal range (70–130 mg/dl) or when blood glucose levels fall below 70 mg/dl (hypoglycemia). For others, irritability or sadness can occur when blood glucose levels are higher (say, above 250 mg/dl). In both cases, changes in mood tend to be temporary and will be reduced or cease when blood glucose returns to your target range.

Find Out More: Another source of changes in mood is diabetes-related distress. This comes from worry, concern, or feelings of stress associated with the daily routine of managing diabetes. We have learned that diabetes distress is associated with more difficulty managing A1C (a measure of average blood glucose over the previous 2–3 months). Talk with your doctor or diabetes educator if you feel that you are struggling with your diabetes. They can help!

Finally, one in four people with type 1 or type 2 diabetes develops long-standing depressive symptoms. This may involve feeling sad, blue, or bored nearly every day, in combination with changes in sleep or appetite, poor concentration, feeling worthless or very guilty about everyday situations, and lack of energy. These symptoms tend to come on gradually and may be associated with life stressors, or they may occur out of the blue but remain for an extended period of time.

If you develop these symptoms, it is important to discuss them with your doctor. Long-standing depression is associated with greater difficulty in managing blood glucose, worsened diabetes complications, and poorer outcomes. The good news is that depression can be effectively treated with medications and/or talk therapy and exercise.

Takeaway: Tell your doctor if you have experienced any of these changes in mood so that you can discuss the options that will work best for you.

Can I Put Diabetes behind Me?

was diagnosed with type 2 diabetes about 10 years ago. Through diet and exercise, I have lost 35 pounds, and I maintain an A1C around 5.7% or less. I've never been on medication, but I feel the need to check my blood glucose daily so as not to relapse. My current doctor says I now don't have diabetes. Can a person with diabetes truly become nondiabetic?

S. Y. C., Portland, OR

Belinda Childs, APRN, MN, BC-ADM, CDE, responds: You ask an interesting question that may not have one right answer. Another way to put your question is: Can type 2 diabetes be cured?

Let's start with what we know about type 2 diabetes. We know that the risk factors for type 2 diabetes include a family history of the disease, older age, being overweight, getting limited physical activity, having had a baby weighing over 9 pounds, and being of certain races and ethnicities, such as African American, Native American, Latino, or Asian. We know that type 2 diabetes in its early phase can be controlled by meal planning, weight loss, and increased exercise, and that these are the cornerstones of diabetes treatment.

Diabetes can now be diagnosed using the A1C (a measure of average blood glucose over the previous 2–3 months), according to American Diabetes Association guidelines. If one has an A1C greater than or equal to 6.5%, the diagnosis is diabetes. If the A1C is between 5.7% and 6.4%, the person is diagnosed with prediabetes and action to prevent diabetes is recommended, including weight loss and increased physical activity. For most people with type 2 diabetes, the treatment goal is for the A1C to be less than 7%, although some people have higher or lower targets.

Most diabetes experts would say that you have controlled, if not cured, your type 2 diabetes through meal planning and exercise. But if you were to regain weight and decrease your physical activity, it is very likely that your blood glucose levels would rise again to their previous levels.

The one instance where type 2 diabetes often appears to go into remission is with gastric bypass weight-loss surgery. This surgery physically reconfigures the digestive tract in a way that may alter the so-called gut hormones. But gastric bypass is generally recommended only for people who are extremely overweight (BMI >35 kg/m^2).

Type 2 diabetes is a result of genetic and environmental influences. We can alter our environmental influences, including what we eat and drink and how much physical activity we get. But we can't change our genetic makeup. And so once a person has had type 2 diabetes, he or she will always have diabetes, or at least be at risk for it, and should continue to be monitored for the complications of diabetes.

Nutrition

2

Does Diet Make a Difference?

O n the American Diabetes Association's type 2 diabetes message board, someone posted the comment: "I do know that 85% of your cholesterol levels are determined not by your diet but by heredity, so while diet can make a difference, the effect on cholesterol is limited."

How would you reply to that? How might I motivate someone asking for help with cholesterol?

T. M., New York, NY

Craig Williams, PharmD, responds: The contribution of diet versus genetics to any given individual's cholesterol levels is something we can't determine with any real accuracy. It is generally true that genetics is more important. However, there is an interaction between the two, and the importance of diet should never be discounted.

Although this is true even in patients who do not become overweight, it is particularly evident in patients who do become overweight or obese. Regardless of the content of the diet, when too many calories result in extra, unwanted pounds, this can have the profoundly negative effects of both increasing total cholesterol and lowering "good" cholesterol (HDL).

In patients who do not become overweight, having an unhealthy diet (high in saturated fats and low in soluble and insoluble fiber) still has a negative impact, namely, it increases "bad" cholesterol (LDL). The extent to which improving diet can improve cholesterol varies, but the effects can be very significant.

The Ornish diet,* which stresses a lot of fruit and vegetables with very low fat intake, has been found to be able to lower cholesterol by nearly 50%. With the more common changes in diet that we see in clinical practice, reductions of 10–20% are more likely. Still, remember that greater changes can produce greater benefits.

It is worth noting that the cardiovascular benefits of a healthy diet go beyond just the changes in cholesterol. A large study published in 2013 found a nearly 30% reduction in heart attacks and strokes from eating a Mediterranean diet,* which emphasizes eating more fruits, vegetables, and whole grains while reducing the intake of meat and full-fat dairy products.

The benefits of a healthier diet can be great even if it doesn't dramatically lower your cholesterol.

*The American Diabetes Association does not endorse a specific diet but suggests following a meal plan that fits your individual needs and goals.

What Are Net Carbs?

I have type 1 diabetes, and my son recently gave me a package of sugar-free hard candy that was labeled "0 net carbs." The back of the package said, "To calculate net carbs, subtract the sugar alcohols from the total carbs in the product, because sugar alcohols have minimal impact on blood glucose." I am concerned and confused about this labeling.

S. W., Gainesville, FL

Madelyn L. Wheeler, MS, RDN, CD, FADA, FAND, responds: The term "net carbs" came about when the low-carb food fad began years ago and companies were seeking a way to market their products as being low in carbohydrate. A food's total carbohydrate count (in grams) is arrived at by subtracting the grams of protein, fat, moisture, and ash (residue from protein and carbohydrate) from the food's total weight. What's left is the total carbohydrate. On a nutrition label, the total carbohydrate count is required by the U.S. Food and Drug Administration (FDA) to include the full amount of grams from sugar alcohols and fiber. However, these sources of carbohydrate have less impact on blood glucose than others because the body converts them to glucose only partially, or not at all. Some food companies started using the term "net carbs" and defined it to mean the total grams of carbohydrate minus the grams of sugar alcohols, fiber, and glycerin. This equation is not entirely accurate, because some of the sugar alcohols and fiber are absorbed by the body. In fact, about half of the grams of sugar alcohols are metabolized to glucose.

The term "net carbs" does not have a legal definition, and it's not used by the FDA or the American Diabetes Association. When you see it on a label, you should read the nutrition facts and ingredient list for more information. If you are on intensive insulin management, count carbs, and/or manage your diabetes with carb-to-insulin ratios, you can:

1. **Check the product's sugar alcohol content.** You can subtract half of the grams of sugar alcohols (their names often end in "tol") from the total carbohydrate grams and count this as the "available carbohydrate" grams for insulin adjustment purposes. However, if erythritol is the only sugar alcohol listed in the ingredient list, subtract all of the grams of sugar alcohol.
2. **Check the fiber content.** Total fiber in foods comprises many different types of natural fiber and manufactured ingredients. These types of fiber may vary in whether they are digested and how they affect blood glucose. If "Insoluble Fiber" (mainly found on high-fiber cereal labels) is listed on the nutrition facts panel under "Total Carbohydrate," you

can subtract all of the insoluble fiber grams from the total carbohydrate grams and use the result as the "available carbohydrate" grams for insulin adjustment purposes.

Can You Put a Number on Carbs?

'd appreciate learning about how many grams of carbohydrate I should eat as a guideline to keep my glucose numbers normal.

L. D.

Jill Weisenberger, MS, RDN, CDE, responds: Carbohydrate affects blood glucose more than fat and protein do in the diet, so it is important to eat an appropriate amount of carbohydrate. If you eat too much at one time, your blood glucose may become elevated shortly after eating. If you take certain kinds of blood glucose–lowering medications, eating too little may cause hypoglycemia (low blood glucose).

What to Know: The proper amount of carbohydrate varies with the person and depends on medications, blood glucose targets, activity level, degree of insulin resistance, and other individual differences. It's best to concentrate on the number of carbohydrate grams you eat at each meal or snack, not just your daily total. Typically, women can eat about 45 grams of carbohydrate or more at each meal. Men, because of their larger size, may achieve normal blood glucose values with 60 or more grams of carbohydrate per meal. It's important to spread your carbohydrate intake over your day. If, for example, you ate very little carbohydrate at lunch and a big plate of spaghetti for dinner, you may experience a low after lunch and high blood glucose after dinner.

Find Out More: The proof is in the numbers. To see if 45 grams of carbohydrate per meal is right for you, measure your blood glucose right before eating a meal containing roughly 45 grams of carbohydrate. Then measure it again 2 hours after the start of your meal. The difference between the numbers is largely the effect of the meal and, in general, should be no more than 40 mg/dl higher than your premeal number. Do these paired measurements a few times at breakfast, lunch, and dinner over several days (weekday and weekend) to take note of patterns. A registered dietitian nutritionist or a certified diabetes educator will be able to help you interpret your results and tweak your meal plan.

Takeaways: Don't fear carbohydrate. Balanced meals created from healthful sources of carbohydrate, protein, and fat provide optimal health and energy levels, satisfy you and keep you feeling full, and help to prevent the complications of diabetes and other health problems. Your provider can help you determine if you need a change in what you eat and/or your medications to reach your blood glucose targets.

What Is a Good Evening Snack?

My mom, who has diabetes, likes having her tea and a snack before bedtime. Is eating a slice of American or cheddar cheese good for her?

L. B., Trumbull, CT

Sue Robbins, RD, CDE, responds: Eating smaller meals and snacks is a very healthy way to eat, especially if you have type 2 diabetes. In type 2 diabetes, the pancreas is not able to produce as much insulin or use insulin as it once did. Smaller portions and snacks—especially when you're eating carbohydrate-containing foods—may help you achieve better blood glucose control.

Unfortunately, many snacks are high in calories, carbohydrate, and fat. Cheese is high in saturated fat. It may not affect your mom's blood glucose, but it may cause an increase in her cholesterol level and weight. Your mom might try eating cheese that has reduced fat or is made from 2% milk. Other snacks that have little or no carbohydrate include raw veggies with low-fat dip, sugar-free popsicles, one egg, or a handful of nuts.

For a nutritious snack with some carbohydrate, your mother might try having a piece of fruit, like a small apple, or 1/2 cup of canned fruit in juice. Combining the fruit with 1/2 cup of cottage cheese or a tablespoon of peanut butter will give her added protein. Protein may increase satiety (the feeling of being full) when she is done.

If your mom is unsure how snacks will fit into her meal plan or if she takes insulin to control her blood glucose, she should check with her diabetes educator or dietitian for assistance.

How Can I Make Veggies Appealing?

recently married a man with type 2 diabetes. He knows he is supposed to "eat healthy," but he doesn't like veggies—I've tried! He will eat potatoes with every meal, or a salad. But that's it! What should I do? If he drank a daily V-8, would it make up for not eating vegetables?

Name Withheld

Cassandra L. Verdi, MPH, RD, responds: I remember when I met my fiancé and he told me his favorite vegetable was a peanut. I knew that I had some work to do! But all it took was a little creativity and a bit of encouragement. Now he actually looks forward to vegetable dishes.

What to Know: A good goal for people with diabetes is to fill half their plate with nonstarchy vegetables such as greens, carrots, and asparagus. Potatoes are a starchy vegetable and are high in carbohydrate, so it's important to keep potato portions smaller.

You can count 100% vegetable juice as a serving of vegetables, but don't use it to replace whole veggies. Juice is less filling, has less fiber, and can be high in sodium. If you do buy it, choose a low-sodium variety.

Possible Solutions: It's great that your husband likes salad. Add some different veggies to make his salads more colorful and nutritious! Try diced red pepper, cucumber, fresh basil, grilled asparagus, beets, or sautéed mushrooms and onions. Complement the veggies with any combination of dried or fresh fruit, toasted nuts, and light dressing.

Steamed veggies can get boring. Instead, try roasting veggies in the oven. It's simple and you'll be amazed at the flavors you discover. Here's how:

1. Lightly coat chopped vegetables with olive oil (just a teaspoon or two can go a long way).
2. Season with pepper, garlic, or other spices.
3. Spread the veggies out in a single layer on a baking sheet and roast in an oven preheated to around 400°F until they begin to brown.

Try other healthy cooking methods such as grilling or lightly sautéing veggies. These methods bring out the natural sweetness that you won't taste when you eat vegetables raw or steamed.

Get creative in adding veggies to meals. Use them in stir-fries and casseroles, or add cooked veggies to spaghetti sauce.

Find Out More: Looking for healthy vegetable recipes and meal ideas? Sign up for the American Diabetes Association's *Recipes for Healthy Living* e-news and you'll get a new set of recipes each month: www.diabetes.org/recipes.

It's free! You can learn more about planning meals and healthy eating with diabetes at www.diabetes.org/food-and-fitness/food. Or you can visit www.diabetesforecast.org/landing-pages/recipes-and-food.html to browse *Diabetes Forecast* recipes.

Why Does Sugar-Free Food Act like a Laxative?

Why does sugar-free food act like a laxative?

J. S. S., Hamilton, NJ

Nina Watson, MSN, RN, CDE, responds: A wide variety of artificial sweeteners are used in sugar-free foods. A number of symptoms have been attributed to the presence of these additives in food, and whether or not you experience those symptoms may depend on your individual sensitivity to different types of sweeteners.

The primary culprits that cause the laxative effect are sugar alcohols, also known as polyols. Sugar alcohols come from plant products such as fruits and berries. They have what is called an osmotic effect. They act much like the concentrated fructose (the form of sugar in fruit) that is found in prunes. The fructose pulls fluid into the gut, and when it's ingested in large amounts, it can result in bloating and diarrhea. Most people can tolerate sugar alcohols only in small amounts. Some of the common ones include mannitol, sorbitol, xylitol, lactitol, and maltitol.

Some of the other sweeteners have been reported anecdotally to cause diarrhea as well, although no scientific studies have found a connection. A sensitivity to or intolerance of artificial sweeteners may produce other symptoms too. If you experience problems with bloating, diarrhea, or other symptoms after consuming artificial sweeteners, you should limit or avoid the foods that contain these products. Also, remember that a sugar-free food item is not necessarily calorie- or carbohydrate-free. Be sure to read the nutrition facts label and consider how that product fits into your daily meal plan.

Should I Start Following a Gluten-Free Diet?

I have had type 1 diabetes for 20 years. In the past, none of my doctors have suggested that I follow a gluten-free diet. My new doctor and pharmacist have both proclaimed the advantages of this kind of diet. Is there any merit to going gluten-free when you have diabetes?

J. M., Gainesville, TX

Madelyn L. Wheeler, MS, RDN, CD, FADA, FAND, responds: There is no scientific evidence that people with type 1 diabetes need to follow a gluten-free diet unless they've been diagnosed with celiac disease. Celiac disease is an autoimmune disorder in which the body's immune system responds to gluten—a protein found in wheat, rye, and barley—by damaging the lining of the small intestine. The treatment for celiac disease is to follow a gluten-free diet.

The advice you've been given recently may be based on a misunderstanding of the scientific literature. There has been some research into the idea that proteins found in milk, wheat, and other foods may play a role in the development of type 1 diabetes. Although the exact cause of type 1 diabetes is unknown, it is thought that, in people who have genes associated with type 1 diabetes, environmental factors such as viruses, toxins, and diet may cause the immune reaction that destroys the insulin-producing β-cells of the pancreas, resulting in diabetes.

Researchers are trying to determine the specific factors that may be involved. They have done animal studies, epidemiological reports (which evaluate existing data on entire groups of people), and a small number of studies on human tissue. So far there is some indication that the gastrointestinal tract, as well as possible dietary antigens such as milk protein or wheat protein, may play a role in the development of type 1 diabetes in people. (An antigen is something the body sees as foreign and tries to destroy by creating an immune response.) However, findings are conflicting and inconclusive. A definitive study would have to be conducted by randomly assigning groups of people to different diets, controlling for any outside variables, and evaluating the people over time to see if they develop diabetes.

Although existing research is thought provoking, the studies don't conclude that people with type 1 diabetes should follow a wheat-free or gluten-free diet. Still, there's no harm in trying it. If you decide to go gluten-free, you should work with a dietitian who is familiar with both diabetes and gluten-free diets to make sure that your goals for nutrition and blood glucose control continue to be met.

What about Celiac Disease?

My celiac disease went undiagnosed until middle age—resulting in major osteoporosis and a lot of damage to my intestinal tract (despite my careful adherence to a gluten-free diet). I still have problems with unpredictable absorption of food.

The amount of insulin I need for the same meal can vary greatly even if all other things are seemingly equal (sleep, exercise, etc.). All the doctors I have asked about celiac disease and diabetes have said they don't know anything about it.

B. G., Wynnewood, PA

Sue Robbins, RD, CDE, responds: Celiac disease is a digestive autoimmune disease that damages the intestines and blocks the absorption of the nutrients in food. The treatment for celiac disease is to remove all sources of gluten, a protein found in barley, rye, and wheat, from the eating plan, including contamination from eating utensils and dishes that have come in contact with gluten-containing foods.

Unfortunately, in your case it appears that you have significant long-term damage to the intestinal tract that may be affecting the absorption of the food that you are eating. Normally, ingested carbohydrate will be absorbed and your blood glucose will start to rise in about 15–20 minutes. Rapid-acting insulin, such as insulin lispro, insulin aspart, or insulin glulisine, will begin working about the same time as the blood glucose begins to rise. If you take your insulin, and you do not absorb the carbohydrate, you are certainly at risk for low blood glucose. I would recommend that you ask your doctor about the possibility of using a continuous glucose monitor, which allows you to know what your blood glucose is at any time and track rapid increases and decreases.

Many people with diabetes, especially type 1 diabetes, have unexplained variability in blood glucose concentrations from time to time, despite identical physiological conditions (which of course we all find very puzzling and frustrating). This could explain at least part of what you are observing.

How Do I Eat with Diabetes and Ulcerative Colitis?

H ow do you deal with dietary requirements for managing diabetes when you are also on a diet for ulcerative colitis? This
means no dairy products, no fresh fruit or vegetables, no
chocolate, etc. Any ideas?

M. L., Woodridge, IL

Sue Robbins, RD, CDE, responds: Ulcerative colitis is difficult to live with, especially if you have diabetes too. Diet and lifestyle may help you control symptoms and prevent flare-ups.

For starters, limit your dairy products, as you mentioned. Many people with ulcerative colitis are lactose intolerant as well. (Lactose is a sugar that is found in milk.) Cheese and yogurt are generally well tolerated because lactose is broken down in the processing. Adding a dietary supplement that helps you break down lactose is another good idea. Foods with fiber may be problematic as well. If fresh fruits and vegetables aggravate symptoms, try cooking, baking, or stewing them. You'll have to try a variety of vegetables because people vary in what their systems will tolerate. Be cautious of vegetables from the cabbage family. These include broccoli, cauliflower, and Brussels sprouts, as well as cabbage.

Legumes, spicy foods, alcohol, and caffeine may be irritating. You should also focus on getting adequate protein. Fat may be problematic for your ul- cerative colitis, though, so focus on lean meats, like skinless chicken, fish, lean ground beef, pork tenderloin, and egg whites.

Eating small meals may be helpful in balancing both dietary issues. And remember to drink plenty of fluids but to be careful with carbonated bever- ages. They may cause gas.

To individualize a meal plan that will work for you and help control both conditions, make an appointment with a registered dietitian. A professional consultation can help expand your choices and your nutrition, especially if your diet is very limited or you are losing weight.

How Should I Eat with Gastroparesis?

was recently diagnosed with gastroparesis, but I'm unclear about what I can and can't eat. Do you have any meal-planning guidelines?

J. L., Redlands, CA

Meghann Moore, RD, CDE, MPH, responds: Gastroparesis can make certain foods more difficult to digest, so it's great that you're thinking in advance about meal planning.

What to Know: Gastroparesis is a complication of diabetes where the nerves and muscles that regulate stomach emptying do not work properly. This can lead to abdominal pain and discomfort with heartburn, fullness and bloating, nausea, and vomiting. Some people also experience constipation, diarrhea, or both. Gastroparesis may affect up to 50% of people with diabetes.

Possible Solutions: There is not a lot of research on nutrition and gastroparesis. Current recommendations are based on what we know about the disease and what patients tell us works for them. When planning meals, look for foods that digest quickly: non-whole-grain breads, cereals, and crackers; peeled soft fruits; well-cooked vegetables (not raw); lean proteins prepared with minimal fat; and juice and milk as tolerated.

Aim to eat six small meals and snacks during the day, with 15–45 grams of carbohydrate each. Liquid foods (beverages, shakes, soups) are more easily digested than solids, and low-fiber foods are best, as fiber can delay stomach emptying. Avoid high-fiber foods such as berries, Brussels sprouts, whole grains, and legumes because of the risk for formation of a bezoar (an indigestible mass of food residue in the stomach).

Eating a high-protein diet or neglecting to chew your food thoroughly can aggravate gastroparesis. Finally, be sure you are getting enough of the nutrients you need each day, especially magnesium, iron and ferritin, vitamin B12, and 25-hydroxy vitamin D; your health-care provider can monitor your lab values of these, and a dietitian can discuss foods that best meet your needs.

Takeaways: Stick to small, frequent meals and snacks with foods that are low to moderate in fat content and low in fiber content. Eat slowly, take small bites of food, and chew your food well. Discuss with your doctor whether any medication changes are needed because of changes in when, what, and how often you eat or because of changes in your absorption of food. Do your best to keep your blood glucose levels in target range day to day, and avoid major glucose swings by keeping your carbohydrate intake moderate and spread out evenly through the day.

Exercise & Weight Loss

3

Can I Exercise with a High Blood Glucose?

've read that it's not good to exercise with a blood glucose of 250 mg/dl or higher. Do you still burn calories when you are this high? Sometimes after exercise I'll test and my blood glucose has gone up, and I wonder if my workout was all for nothing.

A. A. B., Minneapolis, MN

Christy Parkin, MSN, RN, CDE, responds: Exercise is an important part of any diabetes treatment plan, and it's a powerful weapon against high blood glucose levels. However, diabetes and exercise pose special challenges, and for many people with diabetes, it's important to test before and after exercise to prevent potentially dangerous blood glucose fluctuations.

The reason you need to be cautious with a blood glucose level of 250 mg/dl or higher is that there may not be enough insulin available to lower the blood glucose. This is especially important in type 1 diabetes, in which the body is insulin deficient and prone to ketones in the absence of insulin. During exercise, the muscles need more energy, so the liver responds by releasing glucose into the bloodstream. If the body does not have enough insulin to help glucose enter muscle and other cells, the glucose remains in the bloodstream. This can cause more frequent urination and lead to dehydration, especially when you lose additional fluid from sweating and breathing hard during exercise. Additionally, if the body is forced to burn excessive amounts of fat for fuel, as is the case when insulin levels are too low, toxic ketones can build up in the blood, and that can lead to diabetic ketoacidosis, a life-threatening condition.

To be safe, it is best to check your ketones with a urine or blood ketone strip when your blood glucose is over 250 mg/dl. This will indicate whether you have enough insulin on board to safely exercise. If ketones are present, hold off exercising until your blood glucose has come down. If there are no ketones present (in both type 1 and type 2 diabetes), then proceed cautiously with your exercise program.

How Do I Control Low Blood Glucose during Exercise?

I have type 2 diabetes and am 53 years old. I am currently taking water aerobics and using the stationary bike and treadmill. But my blood glucose drops drastically after about 15–20 minutes of heavy cardio exercise. There is no way I can lose weight with this problem, because I have to eat every time I exercise to bring my glucose level up. Any ideas?

T. N., Missouri City, TX

Janis McWilliams, RN, MSN, CDE, BC-ADM, responds: What you describe is very frustrating and can be an issue for people with diabetes trying to increase their activity. An exercise regimen will improve cardiovascular fitness, but hopes of weight loss seem sabotaged by having to "feed" the low blood glucoses with fast-acting carbohydrate sources such as juice or glucose tablets. The key to avoiding this is to appropriately plan for the increased activity.

Exercise is an important part of diabetes management, and has been shown to improve blood glucose control, reduce heart disease risk factors, help with weight loss, and improve well-being. The American Diabetes Association recommends at least 150 minutes of moderate-intensity exercise per week, but you should check with your provider first, especially if you have issues like what you are describing. You may need to have your medication doses reduced or switch to a medication that doesn't cause hypoglycemia. Checking your blood glucose before exercise is always a good idea, and if your levels are below 100 mg/dl, then you should eat or drink something that contains 15 grams of carbohydrate and recheck your blood glucose. Always have a fast-acting carbohydrate with you when you exercise. Protein will not help bring up your blood glucose during exercise.

When people use multiple daily insulin injections or are using an insulin pump, it is easy to reduce the amount of rapid-acting (mealtime) insulin prior to exercise. Sometimes doses of long-acting insulin or the basal rate of pumped insulin are also reduced on exercise days. The decision of how much the dose should be reduced and over what time period is based on the timing and type of exercise and the insulin treatment plan. Check with your provider about these adjustments. Insulin users should avoid injecting, before exercise, into a limb they will be actively using. It is not as easy to adjust oral medication, but if you are on a sulfonylurea (such as glipizide or glyburide), talk with your provider about taking a lower dose on exercise days.

You did not say what time of the day you typically exercise, but you might try timing your exercise to 1–2 hours after a meal, when your glucose will typically be increased. It is also a good idea to learn when your medication is working at its best, or its "peak." Since you have had problems with hypoglycemia, try scheduling your exercise for a time of day that avoids this peak. You can ask your pharmacist for the time(s) when your particular medications peak.

Finally, be aware that hypoglycemia can occur during or long after exercise. Check your blood glucose throughout the day and during the night to see if you are prone to delayed hypoglycemia. Having a balanced postworkout snack can help to stabilize your glucose and prevent hypoglycemia after vigorous exercise.

Check with your health-care provider before making any medication changes. You may also want to talk to a diabetes educator, who can work with you to incorporate physical activity into your daily routine.

Too Much Exercise?

have type 2 diabetes, and my A1Cs are usually around 6.2%.
I recently started exercising more. At first, my blood glucose
was low all day. But now, with the same amount of food, meds,
etc., my A1C is 6.4%. I'm in better shape, but how can I get my
numbers lower?

P. T., Tallmadge, OH

Christy Parkin, MSN, RN, CDE, responds: You can think of exercise as a great
blood glucose–lowering drug—most of the time. In some cases, blood glucose
can temporarily increase with exercise. But the healthful effects of exercise are
much longer lasting and worth the effort.

What to Know: When exercising, the body needs extra energy (in the form
of glucose) for the muscles. For short bursts, such as a quick run across the
street, the muscles and liver release stores of glucose for fuel. With continued
moderate exercising, though, your muscles take up glucose at almost 20 times
the normal rate. This lowers blood glucose levels.

However, if not enough insulin is present (beginning at blood glucose levels of 250 to 300 mg/dl), exercise can result in a rise in blood glucose. In addition, prolonged or strenuous exercise can cause your body to produce adrenaline and other hormones that can cause your blood glucose to rise temporarily.

Possible Solutions: Seeing how you respond to exercise involves trial and
error. Some people report blood glucose spikes with morning exercise, but not
in the evening. Because blood glucose often rises at first after exercise, consider waiting at least an hour to check your blood glucose to give your body a
chance to recover and settle down after exercise.

Takeaways: Although your A1C level went up slightly, the rise was within
normal levels of lab variations. Congratulate yourself on your blood glucose
control and on being in better shape, and continue to exercise. Longer periods
of moderate exercise may help lower your numbers to target as you use your
body's insulin more efficiently; if not, the progressive nature of type 2 diabetes
may require medication adjustments.

How Can I Exercise with Physical Disabilities?

I was born with multiple birth defects, including curvature of the spine, a dislocated hip, and clubfeet. Fifteen years ago I was diagnosed with type 2 diabetes. I also have congestive lung disease and congestive heart failure. With all this, I cannot walk more than 150 feet without getting out of breath. My legs and feet are constantly swollen. How do I exercise?

R. L. R., Hazle Township, PA

Bret Goodpaster, PhD, responds: The short answer to your question is that, as you have already experienced, traditional exercise will be a major challenge. Your disabilities preclude you from performing some of the most common types of exercises. You definitely should consult with your own doctor and with a physical therapist or exercise physiologist who can assess in person exactly which exercises will work for you.

In general, these might include arm or upper-body exercises, such as those with light hand weights or weight machines. You might also try swimming or water exercises, but be sure to exercise in the presence of a lifeguard or swimming instructor who can help you if you need it.

Many patients with diabetes have physical limitations, such as neuropathy, that might keep them from walking for extended periods of time. Still, there are various activities that may be worked into an exercise regimen, even if their duration or intensity must be limited. These exercises might include shorter periods of walking, stationary cycling, rowing, and swimming.

Physicians, nurses, and many diabetes educators may not have the appropriate training to provide guidance about exercise for special conditions or limitations. So it is particularly important for you to get help from the right professionals. You may need to ask your doctor to refer you to a physical therapist or an exercise physiologist. Call your insurance company and ask what is covered; don't be surprised if you're told that you'll have to pay for some or all of these services out of pocket. But don't hesitate to reach out; exercise is vital to diabetes management, and lack of exercise can only exacerbate physical limitations or, worse, lead to further disabilities.

How Do I Persuade My Spouse to Lose Weight?

My husband is so overweight. How can I persuade him to lose weight? I have tried everything!

Name Withheld

Paul Ciechanowski, MD, MPH, responds: Instead of asking how you can persuade your husband to lose weight, a better question is: How can you create the circumstances to help him reach this goal? As a caring family member, you may be uniquely positioned to help him in several ways.

Direct persuasion on your part may backfire if your husband is not already motivated to change. He may feel that you are trying to control him, which will make him resist your help even more. In order to create the circumstances for change, ask yourself these questions:

- What are his views and perceptions about his weight?
- Does he think he needs to lose weight?
- How aware is he of the health risks of being overweight? Does he already have diabetes, heart disease, high blood pressure, and/or high cholesterol?
- If he wants to lose weight, does he have the tools to succeed? For example, has he ever been physically active on a regular basis? Or does he lack the confidence to engage in regular exercise? Does he have experience regulating his own diet and eating nutritious foods, or is this something he will have to learn about?

The best way to support your husband may not be through examining his habits alone, but by examining your household approach to physical activity and healthy eating. You might try:

- Stocking up on nourishing foods like whole grains, fruits, and vegetables, and lean protein sources.
- Limiting the availability of high-calorie snacks and desserts.
- Beginning to take regular walks as a couple or as a family.
- Joining an activity center, gym, or community center, or engaging in active group programs as a couple.
- Getting a pet. Research shows that having a dog increases the likelihood of regular walking.

These suggestions will not be a solution for everyone. Many times, people who are dealing with an overwhelming schedule, or shame about their weight, may not have success resolving the issue despite the encouragement of loved ones. Physical or mental health conditions can also be barriers to weight loss. Your husband may want to get screened for stress, anxiety, and depression.

These are often accompanied by emotional eating and lack of motivation, which are also associated with weight gain.

Finally, remember that you have special insight into the obstacles your husband faces in trying to lose weight (like long hours at work or joint pain). Consider what reasons there are for your husband not to change his behavior. Understanding what's keeping him overweight may help you both.

How Do I Keep My Blood Glucose Down and My Weight Steady?

I have lost enough weight but continue to keep losing. What can I eat that won't make my blood glucose go higher but will help me maintain my weight?

J. F., Baltimore, MD

Madelyn L. Wheeler, MS, RDN, CD, FADA, FAND, responds: Congratulations on your weight-loss accomplishments! Your first step should be to have a meeting with your dietitian and other members of your diabetes team to adjust your meal plan, and perhaps your diabetes medications, while keeping up your level of physical activity.

Maintaining your weight after losing pounds will generally involve two steps: modestly increasing your caloric intake, and establishing which foods you can choose from in adding those calories. This will depend on what diabetes and other medications you take, how many calories you consume daily, your meal pattern, your exercise plan, and more.

In general, if you are losing about 1 pound every 2 weeks, and if you are consistent in following your meal plan, recommended calorie intake, and physical activity, then adding 250 calories per day to your meal plan should stabilize your weight.

These calories could come from fish and poultry, lean meats, lower-fat cheeses, nuts, nonstarchy vegetables, and whole-grain and fiber-rich starchy foods. Do not add the calories in the form of sweets, desserts, caloric beverages, added sugars, or foods that are high in saturated fats. And instead of eating all the additional calories at one meal, divide them evenly among the meals and snacks you currently have throughout the day. You might want to refer to the American Diabetes Association's booklet *Choose Your Foods: Food Choices for Diabetes*, which can help you choose food serving sizes and calorie values that are equivalent to the number of calories you're trying to add.

Finally, be sure to keep watching food portion sizes and to continue your exercise program. Routinely checking and keeping track of your weight may also help prevent eventual weight regain.

Why Don't I Lose More Weight?

I used to weigh around 300 pounds (in early 2010), and I got down to 223, with an A1C of 5.1% (mid-2011). Now I weigh 240 pounds, with my A1C at 5.3%. I eat around 40 grams of carbohydrate per meal and 1,200 to 1,400 calories per day. But I struggle to lose weight. Am I not eating enough?

N. Y.

Cassandra L. Verdi, MPH, RD, responds: Weight regain is common among people who have lost a lot of pounds. Weight maintenance is very complex and something that many people struggle with. Here are a few things to consider in assessing your situation.

Possible Solutions: Take a look at how much exercise you're doing. Exercise is important not only for weight loss but also for preventing weight regain. According to the American College of Sports Medicine, most people need at least 250 minutes per week of moderate-intensity exercise to maintain weight loss. That comes to nearly an hour of exercise, 5 days per week.

It's great that you're keeping close track of the carbohydrate you eat, which is a key strategy for blood glucose control. But your portions of noncarbohydrate foods may have gotten larger over time. It's easy for extra calories to slip in, so try keeping a food diary for a week. Write down everything that you eat, measure portion sizes, and record calorie intake. At week's end, study the diary to see where extra calories may be sneaking in.

Your calorie needs depend on your height, weight, age, sex, and other factors. Based on your weight, 1,200 to 1,400 calories per day may not be enough for you. When you consume fewer calories, your body's metabolism adjusts to that new lower calorie level. It could be that your metabolism is being suppressed because you are not eating enough.

Find Out More: The American Diabetes Association has tools that can help. For basic guidance about exercise, a good place to start is www.diabetes.org/food-and-fitness/fitness. For tracking meals, try MyFoodAdvisor at tracker.diabetes.org.

Takeaway: If keeping a food diary and increasing your activity level don't help, you may want to ask your primary care physician for a referral to a registered dietitian (RD) who can develop a weight-loss plan that works for you.

Will Weight-Loss Surgery Help?

I have had type 2 diabetes for 15 years and started insulin therapy 2 years ago. I plan to have bariatric surgery. Is it likely to cause my diabetes to go into remission after I've had the disease for so long?

Name Withheld

Alison B. Evert, MS, RD, CDE, responds: As the twin epidemics of obesity and type 2 diabetes continue to worsen, there is increasing interest in bariatric surgery for weight loss and blood glucose control.

What to Know: Despite what is commonly reported in the news, diabetes is not cured by bariatric surgery. However, the surgery may result in the remission—normalized blood glucose levels with no need for medication—of type 2 diabetes (but not type 1 diabetes) in about 40–95% of cases. People who have higher A1Cs, use insulin, and have had diabetes longer may have a reduced likelihood of remission.

There are two major classes of bariatric surgery: gastric bypass and adjustable gastric banding procedures. Gastric bypass procedures restructure the digestive system; they include "Roux-en-Y" gastric bypass, vertical sleeve gastrectomy, biliopancreatic diversion, and biliopancreatic diversion with duodenal switch. Adjustable gastric banding procedures are less invasive. Gastric bypass results in more weight loss and higher rates of diabetes remission than adjustable banding. The Roux-en-Y gastric bypass is by far the most commonly performed procedure. However, the vertical sleeve gastrectomy is now gaining popularity.

Find Out More: You will want to carefully weigh the risks and benefits of weight-loss surgery, including your chances of diabetes remission, with your health-care team. Although bariatric surgery is at present the most effective therapy to combat severe obesity, it, like any surgical procedure, is not without risks.

Takeaways: Even if you do not have complete remission, bariatric surgery can offer major improvements in glucose control, in addition to weight loss. The long-term benefit of improved glucose control may be the reduction of diabetes complications. Many people who do not experience remission of diabetes following bariatric surgery still may be able to reduce blood glucose medications. Medical and supportive care after surgery is very important to reduce the risk of weight regain and complications such as vitamin and mineral deficiencies, osteoporosis, and rare—but often severe—episodes of hypoglycemia. Research studies need to be performed that compare the long-term benefits, cost-effectiveness, and risks of bariatric surgery in individuals with type 2 diabetes with the benefits and risks of intensive lifestyle and medical interventions.

Is Gastric Bypass a Cure?

've heard that people who have gastric bypass surgery "lose" their diabetes almost immediately. I've also heard that many of those who have had gastric bypass regain some of their weight after a while. When this happens, does the diabetes reoccur?

Name Withheld

Robert A. Gabbay, MD, PhD, responds: Gastric bypass helps some people with type 2 diabetes in a number of ways. Clearly, the profound weight loss that many people experience after this kind of surgery helps their diabetes by improving blood glucose, cholesterol, and blood pressure. What is interesting is that some of the benefits—in particular, the improvement in blood glucose control—happen very quickly after the surgery, before much weight loss has occurred. It is believed that by bypassing some of the intestine, hormones from the gut are changed, improving the body's ability to make insulin. After gastric bypass surgery, many people have been able to—in consultation with their health-care providers—stop some of their diabetes medications. Some people are even able to stop all diabetes medications. In some ways, this might be called a "cure," but in other ways, we are not sure yet.

Health-care providers often consider that the diabetes these people have—the people who are able to stop taking diabetes medications after surgery—is being controlled through weight loss. But the reason it is important to not consider this a true "cure" is that these people still need to be periodically evaluated for diabetes complications. Despite stopping diabetes medications, people who have undergone gastric bypass should still continue their screenings and preventive measures, including having their eyes examined annually and having their urine checked for protein and kidney disease. Some people do regain some of the weight lost after surgery, and for them, the need for medications to treat their diabetes often returns.

Should I Test My Blood Glucose?

I was diagnosed with type 2 diabetes 16 years ago. Over these years, I have been a patient at a local medical practice. Because of staff turnover, I've had three different physicians in that time. All three have discouraged home testing, saying that the A1C test is far superior. They have shown no interest in my own finger-stick test results.

I have my A1C test, followed by an appointment with my doctor, quarterly. My blood glucose is well controlled and I am not overweight. I have none of the classic diabetes symptoms. I have gone from testing daily, to testing occasionally, to testing rarely.

Should I be testing regularly, even though my doctors don't believe in it and don't want to know the results?

W. C., North Wales, PA

Paris Roach, MD, responds: The frequency with which you should monitor your blood glucose will depend on how you plan to use the information. People who take multiple daily doses of insulin or use insulin pumps need to monitor at least three to four times (sometimes as many as six to eight times) daily to stay safe and to adjust insulin doses for high or low glucose levels. Those not on insulin but who are in the process of having their medications adjusted should monitor often enough to guide the medication adjustments, usually two to three times a day. If you're on medications that can cause hypoglycemia, like sulfonylureas (such as glipizide or glyburide), you should have a working blood glucose meter and test strips on hand so you can conduct a blood glucose check if you feel low, if you're planning to engage in physical activity or drive, or if you have to miss or delay a meal.

Even if you're not on a medication that can cause hypoglycemia, and have achieved your glucose control targets, it may be a good idea to perform spot checks of your glucose at least a few times a week for your own information. You should also perform a "glucose profile" (checking your blood glucose before and 2 hours after each meal) once or twice every month or so to see if your glucose patterns are changing over time. This information can help you double-check the general accuracy of your A1C test results (the measure of your average blood glucose for the previous 2–3 months). You should check your blood glucose more frequently if you experience an illness or if you have symptoms that you think may be related to your blood glucose level.

What Affects My Blood Glucose?

I have type 2 diabetes, and my A1C is about 6%. I really don't understand how caloric intake affects my blood glucose. Suppose that I ate a meal of meat, potato, vegetable, apple pie, and milk, in quantities that I got 100 calories from each. Would each contribute an equal amount to my blood glucose?

B. C., Missoula, MT

Madelyn L. Wheeler, MS, RDN, CD, FADA, FAND, responds: Blood glucose comes mainly from the carbohydrate in food you eat (it's also affected by how physically active you are). Your body breaks the carbohydrate down into glucose, which supplies you with energy or is stored as fat. The hormone insulin helps usher glucose into the cells. Having type 2 diabetes usually means that your body doesn't respond properly to insulin, produce enough insulin, or both.

In the meal you describe, 100 calories from each of the five foods would not affect your after-meal blood glucose equally because their carb content differs. Plain meat, fish, poultry, and fats such as margarine or butter do not contain carbohydrate. The other food groups (starches, nonstarchy and starchy vegetables, fruits, milk and other dairy products such as yogurt, and other "combination" foods such as desserts) all contain carbohydrate.

The table below shows the weight or volume and carb content for 100 calories of each of the five foods.

Food	Weight/ Volume	Carbohydrate (grams)	Calories
Meat (hamburger, 96% lean)	2 oz	0	100
Potato (boiled plain)	2/3 cup	23	100
Nonstarchy Vegetable (green beans)	2 1/2 cups	23	100
Apple Pie	1 1/3 oz	14	100
Milk (nonfat)	1 1/4 cups	15	100

As you can see, it takes 2 1/2 cups of a nonstarchy vegetable like green beans to total 100 calories, much more than a starchy potato, even though both have 23 grams of carbohydrate. Green beans have a low calorie (energy) density. They contain a lot of water and so are very filling. Apple pie, which is packed with fat and sugars, has a high calorie density. Just a small amount produces many calories.

A healthy meal plan will include a variety of foods. If you are overweight, counting calories may help with shedding pounds. Losing weight can help your body use insulin more effectively and improve blood glucose control. That, in turn, helps you avoid diabetes complications. Your A1C is evidence of good blood glucose control; congratulations for keeping it on target.

Why Does Blood Glucose Go Up Some Days and Not Others?

W hy does my wife's blood glucose go up to 230 mg/dl at dinnertime (5 p.m.) on some days, while on other days that doesn't happen even though she eats about the same food? My wife has type 2 diabetes.

Name Withheld

Janis McWilliams, RN, MSN, CDE, BC-ADM, responds: Even minor changes in meals, physical activity, and overall health can affect blood glucose.

Carbohydrate in foods causes a person's blood glucose to rise. However, different types of carbohydrate-containing foods can have varying impacts on how quickly and how much blood glucose goes up. In addition, the amount of fat and fiber in these foods can slow your body's absorption of the carbohydrate, making your number appear lower after eating than it typically would, but higher a few hours later.

What you eat is only one factor that can affect blood glucose. Medications can have an effect on your glucose. Some medications, such as steroids, can raise it. If you are using insulin, your injection site can affect how the insulin is absorbed. That can change the action of the insulin in bringing down your blood glucose. And if you take your medications late or not at all, that can also have an effect.

Stress can contribute to high blood glucose. The body's normal response to stress—both physical and emotional—is to release glucose stored in the liver into the bloodstream. In people with diabetes, this response is exaggerated, and blood glucose levels rise even higher. High blood glucose can also be caused by infection, and you can have an infection without experiencing any other symptoms.

Sometimes, people with diabetes and their health-care providers just can't determine the cause of high blood glucose. This is frustrating for everyone, and you need to remember not to get too upset about one high number, but to focus instead on overall control. Look for patterns and try to determine what might be causing high blood glucose. You can use a logbook, memory features on a blood glucose meter, or diabetes management software to help you look for trends. Include not only your blood glucose values in your record keeping, but also the time you tested, what you ate, when you took your medications, and any other notes from the day. There are also a number of smartphone apps available that you can use to track your blood glucose levels and the foods you eat. Review your log regularly with your doctor or diabetes educator.

Can My "Normal" Be High?

f my blood glucose numbers dip below 120 mg/dl, I start to feel light-headed, and when they get down to 100 or below, I am dizzy. Is it possible that my "normal" numbers should be higher than the recommended low 100s?

Name Withheld

Christy Parkin, MSN, RN, CDE, responds: According to the American Diabetes Association, the recommended fasting blood glucose for people with diabetes is 70–130 mg/dl. After meals, blood glucose should be less than 180 mg/dl. When blood glucose falls below 70 mg/dl, that is considered hypoglycemia, or low blood glucose. Hypoglycemia is common in people with diabetes who take insulin and some oral diabetes medications. Conditions that can lead to hypoglycemia include taking too much medication, missing or delaying a meal, eating too little food for the amount of insulin taken, exercising too strenuously, drinking too much alcohol, or any combination of these factors. Light-headedness is one symptom of low blood glucose; others include shakiness, anxiety, sweating, irritability, clamminess, and rapid heart rate.

Some people with diabetes develop symptoms of low blood glucose at slightly higher levels. If your blood glucose is high for long periods of time, you may have symptoms and feel low when your level is closer to 100 mg/dl. You can also experience hypoglycemic symptoms at normal levels when your blood glucose drops rapidly. Getting your blood glucose under better control can help to lower the level at which you begin to feel symptoms. In other words, you may have to work at "readjusting your thermostat" to get used to lower, more normal blood glucose levels. As you acclimate to the lower blood glucose levels, you will feel more comfortable between 70 and 100 mg/dl.

When possible, you should confirm that you have hypoglycemia by testing your blood glucose with your meter. In general, it is advisable to treat hypoglycemia by consuming 15 grams of fast-acting carbohydrate when your blood glucose falls below 70 mg/dl, or eat your meal if it's time for one. Check glucose again in 15 minutes to make sure it is on the rise.

Consult your health-care providers for individual guidelines on the target blood glucose ranges that are best for you. The lowest safe blood glucose level for a person varies depending on age, medical condition, and ability to sense hypoglycemic symptoms. A target range that is safe for a young adult with no diabetes complications, for example, may be too low for a young child or an older person with other medical problems. In the end, prevention is the best "treatment" for low blood glucose reactions.

How Do I Quickly Bring Down My Blood Glucose?

f you get a high reading when checking your blood glucose, is there a way to get the number down quickly?

Name Withheld

Christy Parkin, MSN, RN, CDE, responds: Before deciding how to treat one episode of high blood glucose, it is important to figure out why the number is high. Some possible causes include eating a large meal, not getting enough physical activity, forgetting to take diabetes medication, and dealing with illness and stress.

Insulin is the medication that will bring blood glucose down the fastest. Someone who uses mealtime insulin can take correction doses to lower blood glucose. This requires a thorough understanding of when to inject, how often to give correction doses, and how much insulin to use. You will need to work with your health-care provider or diabetes educator to learn how to do this.

Apart from administering insulin, another way to lower your blood glucose is to engage in physical activity. Exercise results in an increased sensitivity to insulin. It causes your muscle cells to take up more glucose, leaving less of it to circulate in your bloodstream during and after the physical activity (which often means a lower blood glucose when you test). Frequent, regular exercise is very important to blood glucose control no matter what type of diabetes you have. Research has shown that it is vital in warding off long-term complications like nerve problems (neuropathy), eye problems (retinopathy), heart disease, and kidney disease (nephropathy). Don't forget to check with a health-care provider, though, before making any major changes to your exercise routine. And if you have type 1 diabetes and your glucose is 250 mg/dl or higher, check for urine or blood ketones. You should not exercise if ketones are present.

Although exercise is a great way to bring down your blood glucose when it is high, remember that physical activity should be a part of your lifestyle, not just a tool for producing one good test result. Getting your recommended periodic A1C tests (a measure of average blood glucose for the previous 2–3 months) will help you and your health-care provider determine whether or not your blood glucose control is on target. And when you use your meter to test at home and at work, be sure to look for patterns in the results. This can help you and your diabetes-care team tell whether you need to adjust your meal plan, medications, exercise, or all three. The most important thing you can do to manage diabetes is to find which strategies will work best to help you achieve your blood glucose goals.

How Can I Avoid
Highs and Lows?

I have type 2 diabetes, and I'm insulin dependent. My A1C has been pretty reasonable, although it has drifted above 7% recently. I try to adjust my diet, exercise routine, and insulin to prevent the highs and lows, but very often my next reading is way different than what I might have expected. My extremely fluctuating blood glucose more often than not results in hyperglycemia. How can I avoid the "rollercoaster"?

J. E., Rockville, MD

Christy Parkin, MSN, RN, CDE, responds: Blood glucose levels that fluctuate wildly up and down are thought to be more dangerous than high blood glucose (hyperglycemia) alone. It is believed that erratic hyperglycemia causes the production of free radicals (highly reactive chemicals that can damage cellular molecules) that lead to damage of the cells (known as oxidative stress). This damage is a predictor of cardiovascular disease in diabetes.

It may be helpful for you to get back to basics with your diabetes management. A1C is generally a good indicator of the risk of diabetic complications; however, it is important to understand that having an A1C that's less than 7% does not necessarily indicate blood glucose control. A1C is simply a measure of average blood glucose levels for the previous 2–3 months, and does not provide the whole picture. That is why blood glucose monitoring is so valuable. As you have noticed, checking your blood glucose after meals can help you to determine whether you took enough insulin, or whether you ate too many carbohydrate grams.

I would suggest meeting with a certified diabetes educator for a review of your plan and getting a nutrition consult with a registered dietitian. Learning how to accurately count carbohydrates and adjust mealtime insulin can greatly improve after-meal spikes. If you take rapid-acting insulin before meals, you should take the injection within 15 minutes before eating. I would take a look at your physical activity as well as any recent weight loss or gain. Also, you may want to evaluate how often you have episodes of low blood glucose (hypoglycemia), because this can lead to hyperglycemia (related to overtreating the lows and hormonal responses).

As you can see, there are many possible reasons for the variability in your blood glucose, and each factor must be considered carefully. You may also want to consider wearing a continuous glucose monitor for several days to see how your blood glucose fluctuates throughout the day and night. Talk to your health-care provider at your next visit about your concerns.

Are Highs after Meals Safe?

am 35 years old and have had type 2 diabetes for 2 years. I take 500 mg of metformin once a day. My A1C is always between 6.3% and 6.7%. I have read that blood glucose levels should be 180 mg/dl or less 1 hour after a meal and 140 mg/dl or less 2 hours after a meal.

Is it okay to have a blood glucose of 200 mg/dl an hour or two after a meal, as long as it does come back down within a reasonable amount of time and my A1C tests keep coming in at a good range?

I like to eat, and I find it hard to stay below 180 mg/dl after meals, but I must be doing something right according to my A1C tests.

J. M., Fremont, OH

Christy Parkin, MSN, RN, CDE, responds: Based on your A1C levels, it sounds like you are doing everything right. Congratulations on your diabetes control. However, you are correct to be concerned about blood glucose levels above 200 mg/dl after meals. Research shows that high blood glucose after meals may have damaging effects on your vascular system. This damage occurs even if your A1C is relatively low. So it is very important that you pay attention to your after-meal blood glucose levels. The American Diabetes Association recommends that blood glucose levels be less than 180 mg/dl 1–2 hours after beginning a meal.

One thing you might consider is eating more frequent meals, but with smaller portions of food at each meal. This will spread out your carbohydrate intake and help reduce glucose "spikes" after meals. Exercise after a meal can also help. I suggest that you talk with your health-care team about lifestyle changes or medications to help you get better control over your postmeal glucose levels. Considering your current level of self-management, any additional changes should not be difficult for you to implement.

How Should I Treat Meals?

've had diabetes for 21 years (and have used insulin for 16 years). What should my blood glucose level be 1–2 hours after eating? Should I inject insulin to lower my level? If the blood glucose of a person without diabetes should be about 120 mg/dl after a meal, isn't it logical that I should strive to keep mine the same?

M. O., Davis, IL

Mary M. Austin, RD, MA, CDE, FAADE, responds: I commend you on your interest in keeping your blood glucose in as "normal" a range as is possible. In people who do not have diabetes, blood glucose usually stays below 140 mg/dl after meals.

What to Know: For people with diabetes, the American Diabetes Association recommends that fasting blood glucose should be maintained in the range of 70–130 mg/dl. One to two hours after the beginning of a meal, blood glucose "peaks" should be below 180 mg/dl. The Association recommends, however, that these guidelines be individualized to the needs of the person with diabetes. The rise and fall of blood glucose after a meal are determined by many factors, including what you ate, how much background insulin you had on board, your physical activity level, the timing of your mealtime insulin dose in relation to your meal, and other factors beyond your control.

Find Out More: The postmeal blood glucose target of 120 mg/dl that you suggest may put you at risk for hypoglycemia because the rapid-acting insulin you take at mealtime continues to be active for about 4 hours. Injecting additional insulin 2 hours after a meal to "improve" your blood glucose could be a hasty response that leads to a dangerous hypoglycemic event. In addition to measuring your glucose level 1–2 hours after the first bite of a meal, it may be useful to make note of the result of your next regularly scheduled blood glucose check—is the level in the comfortable 70–130 mg/dl range by then?

Takeaway: I would recommend discussing with your health-care provider your blood glucose monitoring results, your current A1C level, and what your personal fasting and postmeal blood glucose targets should be to keep you in a healthy and safe range while also avoiding hypoglycemia.

What Is Causing My Unexplained High Blood Glucose?

How many people with type 2 diabetes are struggling with high fasting glucose in the morning after values appear normal at bedtime? What explains this fluctuation? What practical actions can people take to normalize their blood glucose levels before noontime?

Also, is there any way to narrow the spread of fasting blood glucose values by taking some action the evening before? What options are available to us besides prescription medications?

J. R., Southfield, MI

Roger P. Austin, MS, RPh, CDE, responds: High fasting blood glucose levels are quite common in people with type 2 diabetes. There are two processes that contribute to this: one is the excessive release of glucose from the liver in people with type 2, and the second is the "dawn phenomenon" of early cortisol release, which occurs as part of the daily wake-up cycle of humans.

First, the liver releases stored glucose at an excessive rate in people with type 2 diabetes. This occurs even when insulin levels are quite high, as in the early stages of the disease. This has been described as "hepatic [liver] resistance to insulin." Type 2 diabetes also includes the progressive loss of insulin production by the pancreas over time. As insulin levels fall, the levels of another hormone, glucagon, rise. Because glucagon stimulates the liver to release stored glucose, fasting blood glucose levels continue to rise.

Everyone, including people who don't have diabetes, experiences the dawn phenomenon to varying degrees. The body produces increased levels of two types of hormones (growth hormone and cortisol) that increase blood glucose levels in people with diabetes. These hormones are released during the night, and the effects are often seen around 4:00 to 5:00 a.m.

Some steps that can be taken to slow down this rise of fasting blood glucose include eating dinner at an earlier time (6:00 or 7:00 p.m. rather than 9:00 or 10:00 p.m.), as well as being physically active early in the evening by doing something like walking or bicycling.

Late evening snacking can also cause increased morning blood glucose levels. For those who are interested, there are a number of very effective medications to treat this condition. These include metformin; incretin mimetics, such as exenatide; long-acting insulins, such as insulin detemir and insulin glargine; and insulin pump therapy.

Why Is My Blood Glucose So High in the Morning?

I am puzzled by my blood glucose pattern. I am not on any medications. My morning fasting blood glucose is always the highest of the day—between 120 and 140 mg/dl. The rest of the day it is in the normal range. Why does this occur?

R. R., Elk Grove, CA

Christy Parkin, MSN, RN, CDE, responds: In the early morning hours, hormonal changes in your body will naturally cause blood glucose to rise. For people who don't have diabetes, the increase in blood glucose is offset by increased insulin production. For people with diabetes, this early morning increase in blood glucose can be a problem.

There are a couple of things going on that make your glucose rise in the morning. One of these is insulin resistance—a condition that means your body's muscle and fat cells are unable to use insulin effectively to lower blood glucose. However, insulin resistance also affects how your liver processes, stores, and releases glucose, particularly at night. The liver is supposed to release small amounts of glucose when you're not eating. But in type 2 diabetes, the liver dumps more glucose than is needed into the bloodstream, especially at night. So, while your hormones are causing a natural rise in blood glucose, your liver is releasing even more glucose into your system. And because your insulin resistance prevents your muscle and fat cells from using the glucose, your blood glucose level rises.

Unlike postprandial (after-meal) blood glucose, which can be somewhat controlled by a meal plan and exercise, high fasting blood glucose usually needs to be treated with medication. Talk to your health-care provider about medications that can help you obtain morning blood glucose levels that are on target.

How Can I Fight
Morning Highs?

M y morning blood glucose is quite elevated (190–260 mg/dl). Is there a certain time before bed that I should eat to help lower my blood glucose? Are there certain foods I should eat after dinner?

N. L.

Belinda Childs, APRN, MN, BC-ADM, CDE, responds: The rise in your blood glucose in the morning may not just be about when you snack at bedtime or what you eat. It may also mean that you need an adjustment in your medications, physical activity, or some combination of all three factors.

What to Know: The dawn effect, or phenomenon, occurs in people with both type 1 and type 2 diabetes. During the night, the body releases wake-up hormones that can make your body's insulin less effective. Meanwhile, the liver releases too much glucose overnight. The result is a rise in blood glucose, which usually occurs sometime between 3:00 and 6:00 a.m.

Find Out More: Recording 3–4 consecutive days of blood glucose levels 3–4 hours after supper or at bedtime and before eating in the morning will allow you and your health-care provider to review how much your blood glucose levels are increasing overnight. A 3:00 a.m. check can also be helpful, as that is around the time when the dawn effect often sets in. This information will help show whether you need a medication change to alter the glucose release or control the rise in blood glucose. It will also provide feedback about any evening snack you may have.

Possible Solutions: Although research does not prove the benefit of a bedtime snack for controlling morning (fasting) blood glucose, many providers still recommend one. The theory is that the food in your system tells your liver to hang on to extra glucose instead of releasing it and raising blood glucose levels. Use your glucose monitoring as a tool to determine the value of a snack for you. A low-fat, high-fiber snack such as air-popped popcorn or reduced-fat string cheese and whole-wheat crackers may be a good choice. Avoid high-fat foods because they can promote insulin resistance and may contribute to morning highs.

Physical activity makes the insulin you make or take work better, and the benefit lasts up to 36 hours. So an afternoon or evening walk is likely to lower your fasting blood glucose the next morning. Finally, talk with your health-care provider to see if you need a change in medication to help control morning highs.

Takeaway: A reminder: the goal for most people with diabetes is fasting blood glucose between 70 and 130 mg/dl.

Why Does My Blood Glucose Vary from One Hand to the Other?

There is always a discrepancy when I test my blood glucose levels on one hand versus the other. This morning I tested my left hand and got a blood glucose reading of 153 mg/dl. I immediately tested my right hand, and it read 167 mg/dl. Why is this happening? Sometimes the difference is as much as 50 mg/dl.

S. L., Columbus, OH

Christy Parkin, MSN, RN, CDE, responds: Blood glucose levels vary from minute to minute, and from body part to body part. It is not unusual to see a difference of plus or minus 15–20% from one reading to another. When meters are reading greater differences, it is time to evaluate other issues such as the integrity of the strips, the cleanliness of the skin, and the technique of obtaining a drop of blood and correctly placing it on the strip.

If you are using a meter that requires coding, make sure that the code is set to match the code on the bottle of strips being used. Since strips are very sensitive to air, moisture, and extreme temperatures, make sure that you re-cap your bottle of strips immediately after taking a strip out. Limit their exposure to light and don't keep them in a cold or hot car or a bathroom with lots of moisture. You can also check your strips using the control solution that may come with your meter.

Sometimes it is helpful to go back to the basics you learned when you first started blood glucose testing. Make sure you wash and dry your hands. Use a lancet device with the shallowest penetration that will get enough blood for the strip that you are using.

If you want to check the accuracy of your meter against a lab value, do a finger stick immediately after your lab draw (you should be fasting). Again, it is acceptable to see a plus or minus 20% variation. Medical conditions to consider are peripheral neuropathy, which can impair circulation, and edema (excess fluid in the tissues), which can also cause blood glucose variations.

It is always a good idea to call the customer service toll-free number on the back of your meter if you have questions and concerns about the accuracy of your meter and strips. Company representatives can help you troubleshoot many of the issues related to your concerns.

Does Altitude Affect Blood Glucose?

I am 72 years old and have had diabetes for 15 years. At sea level in Southern California, with a moderate activity level and normal eating habits, I need between 140 and 150 units of Humalog each day. When I exercise, my blood glucose rises, and I need insulin to come back down. I keep my blood glucose in check by measuring four to six times per day, and I use both a needle and a pump. I control to between 70 and 110 mg/dl and have an A1C of 6.2%.

I currently live in Aspen/Snowmass, Colorado, at an altitude of 8,200 feet. Although I do exercise more, my insulin requirement is between 40 and 50 units each day. In addition, when I exercise, my blood glucose drops, so I can only ski or bike starting at an elevated blood glucose level. Quite the opposite from sea level.

The dawn phenomenon that I experience requires me to take an additional 15 units of insulin at sea level, but only an additional 6 units when I am at a higher altitude.

I have not found an explanation yet for this phenomenon.

W. M., Aspen/Snowmass, CO

Henry Rodriguez, MD, responds: It sounds like the increase in exercise that you engage in when at a higher altitude in Colorado is the major factor causing the decrease in your insulin requirement. In children's diabetes camps, I've seen that a cut of 20% to sometimes 50% of kids' normal insulin doses is required to address the physical activity of camp, depending on the child's usual activity at home. At a higher altitude, the heart rate is higher and insulin may, theoretically, be absorbed more rapidly. My colleague H. Peter Chase, MD, professor of pediatrics at the Barbara Davis Center for Childhood Diabetes at the University of Colorado, assists in a pediatric diabetes camp located in Colorado at an altitude of about 8,500 feet. He has observed similar effects in the children who attend. The medical staff has to decrease everyone's insulin dosages by 20%. Again, this is largely due to the children's increased activity level at camp compared with at home. Over time, we would expect the more modest effect of altitude to lessen as the body adjusts to the elevation.

Is My Blood Glucose Control "Too Good"?

A few months ago, I was advised by a diabetes specialist that my blood glucose control was "too good." My A1C has been between 5% and 5.5% for the past 5 years. My specialist said I should be somewhere between 6.5% and 7%. How does this match up with American Diabetes Association recommendations?

M. B., Wabasha, MN

M. Sue Kirkman, MD, responds: The American Diabetes Association recommends an A1C target of less than 7% for most adults with diabetes, but also advises that treatment goals should be individualized. There is a lot of evidence that glucose control to near-normal levels helps prevent or delay the small-vessel complications of diabetes, such as kidney or eye disease. However, glucose control may not have much impact once complications are advanced, such as when someone is blind from retinopathy. Also, a person with a life expectancy of only a few years (because of advanced cancer, for example) is unlikely to benefit much from tight control, so the A1C target could be relaxed in that case.

Whether good glucose control helps prevent heart attacks or strokes is a more difficult question. Several large studies suggest that it might not, although others propose that if a person practices good glucose control starting soon after diagnosis, it may reduce the rate of heart attacks and of deaths from heart disease 10 or 20 years later. One of the large studies of type 2 diabetes and cardiovascular complications, the ACCORD trial, compared intensive glucose control (a target A1C under 6%) with standard glucose control (a target A1C between 7% and 8%) in people with diabetes. Surprisingly, the mortality rate was highest in the intensive group. Several other large studies of type 2 diabetes have not shown this, so it has been difficult to determine what accounted for the ACCORD results.

Another factor that may affect how tightly you control your blood glucose is your risk for hypoglycemia (low blood glucose). People who take insulin or certain oral medications, like glyburide, are at the highest risk. If your low A1C can be partially attributed to episodes of hypoglycemia, then your health-care provider would most likely advise you to relax your glucose control targets.

Your A1C level has been in the normal range and stable for years. Whether your A1C needs to be "raised" really depends on how you are doing overall, and may be affected by things like hypoglycemia, complications you're experiencing, or other medical conditions. You may have really good glucose control due to a healthy diet and exercise regimen, in which case there seems to be no reason for concern. You and the diabetes specialist who made this recommendation should talk more about what targets make sense for you.

Is Plasma Glucose a Better Measure?

When I changed blood glucose meters, the readings were quite different. The company that makes my new meter says it uses a better system based on plasma glucose instead of whole blood. The readings from plasma seem much higher. Is there an exact differential? Is one system better?

J. V., Canal Winchester, OH

Roger P. Austin, MS, RPh, CDE, responds: You have raised an important issue that is often a cause of confusion for people with diabetes who regularly check their blood glucose levels using blood glucose meters.

What to Know: Glucose can be measured in whole blood, plasma, or serum. In the past, hospital laboratories reported blood glucose values in terms of whole blood, but now they more commonly report plasma glucose values. Plasma has a higher water content than whole blood, so there is more dissolved glucose in plasma compared with whole blood, and readings are 15–20% higher. New blood glucose meters for home use now report blood glucose only in terms of plasma glucose to conform with lab readings.

Possible Solutions: Each manufacturer's blood glucose testing method uses different technology. One is not necessarily better than another—consistency in your checks is what really counts. So, be sure that you use the same meter as much as possible when you check and record your blood glucose readings. Some people may use one meter at home and a different one at the office. Comparing blood glucose results from two or more meters is like comparing apples and oranges; they are not equivalent.

Takeaways: You can take other steps to improve the accuracy of your blood glucose readings. Store meters and strips where they won't be exposed to extremes in temperature or humidity. Before taking a reading, thoroughly wash your hands with soap and warm water (alcohol is not necessary), and dry with a clean towel. Food residue, creams, lotions, or perfumes on your fingers can affect your reading. Finally, know that a finger-stick check, although very useful, is a "snapshot" of your glucose level, which may change quickly.

Are Meters Accurate Enough?

M ore accurate blood glucose meters would help all of us. The manufacturer of my meter says that if the meter gives a reading that is within 20%, it is working fine. This means that if the true reading is 100 mg/dl, I could get results ranging from 80 to 120 mg/dl and the meter is working fine.

Are there reasons for this inaccuracy? Has anyone tried to make them better?

K. D. S., Broadview Heights, OH

David E. Bruns, MD, responds: These are concerns with all medical testing: How accurate are the methods that are available? How accurate must the methods be to meet clinical needs? Both questions are unavoidable because all methods of measurement have error. Both questions are difficult to answer, especially in the case of blood glucose meters.

Many studies have attempted to evaluate the accuracy of blood glucose meters, but many, if not most, of the studies suffer from deficiencies. For example, many papers report the performance of a meter only in the hands of a single highly skilled medical technologist, working under ideal conditions, often paid by the manufacturer (directly or indirectly), sampling a few strips and meters. Such a study does not tell us how the meters perform in the hands of people who are not highly trained medical technologists and who will be doing the testing day or night, under less-than-ideal conditions, potentially with distractions, vision problems, and other challenges. Some of the better studies do address this question, and find that meters do not perform as well under real-life conditions as in laboratories.

Having said that, however, it is also clear that meters have improved over time. Many of the innovations in meters can be expected to make the quality of results less dependent on the environment and on the operator's skill. Such improvements include no-wipe strips, automatic timing, automatic detection of sample volume, and small sample size.

It is difficult to define how well meters perform and how accurate they need to be. We can probably all agree that it would not matter much if a meter reported a result of 99 mg/dl as 100 mg/dl. In contrast, we surely would agree that it would be terrible if a meter reported a glucose of 25 mg/dl as 100 mg/dl. Somewhere between such extremes we must find where an error makes a difference. Despite questions about accuracy, it is clear that the use of glucose meters, even the earliest versions, has had a profound impact on blood glucose control.

Why Not Compare Meters' Accuracy?

Manufacturers of blood glucose meters and diabetes organizations seem reluctant to provide a ranking of the various meters' accuracy. Why? I might even pay more for a meter that exceeded the minimum standard.

T. T., Cedar Park, TX

M. Sue Kirkman, MD, responds: The American Diabetes Association has a long-standing interest in the accuracy of home blood glucose meters and is part of coalitions that are advocating for strengthening international and U.S. Food and Drug Administration (FDA) standards for accuracy. It looks as if the requirements will tighten up in the near future, which can only be good news for people with diabetes, although we don't yet know what the final recommendations will be.

The American Diabetes Association would love to be able to provide comparisons of meters' accuracy for its readers, but there are a number of reasons why it cannot do so. It is a nonprofit organization without a laboratory or expertise in laboratory comparisons of products. Such testing would be very complicated (as a meter company executive explains below) and beyond the Association's capabilities. *Consumer Reports*, the magazine of an organization that does have expertise in rating products, ranked 17 common blood glucose meters in its November 2011 issue. The article says that the meters were compared with "a standard laboratory analyzer," but it doesn't otherwise provide details of the methods used. *Consumer Reports* ranked eight meters as "excellent" for accuracy, six as "very good," and three as "good," and noted that all the meters were well within the current standards for accuracy.

Companies that sell meters in the United States are required to describe their accuracy under "Performance Characteristics" in the package insert that comes with test strips and in the meter's instruction manual. Check the website for the meter brand, and call the customer service line if necessary.

However, even with this information, a comparison among meters is difficult because the results aren't reported in the same way for each meter. Some companies report their accuracy results as a "regression line," with a correlation coefficient, slope, and y-axis. (Yikes! Shades of forgotten algebra!) Other companies report in a table format the percentage of readings above 75 mg/dl that are within plus or minus 5%, plus or minus 10%, and so on. It would be difficult to compare one regression line with another, and even more difficult to compare a regression line to a table. One requirement we'd love to see from the FDA is that all meter companies report their accuracy in the same user-friendly format in their package inserts.

We asked David A. Simmons, MD, of Bayer Diabetes Care to respond to your inquiry, and we appreciate his response below.

David A. Simmons, MD, VP, Head of Global Medical and Clinical Affairs at Bayer Diabetes Care, responds: Thank you for your important question. I agree that people with diabetes should be able to review comparative, head-to-head data related to the devices they must use every day to manage their blood glucose.

Although this sounds like a simple proposition, it actually isn't. In order for a comparison between two devices to be fair and honest, a test would need to be done with each meter using the identical sample of blood, and compared with a reference value (laboratory standard) using the same sample. There are many factors that can affect the results of the test: the blood sample (finger stick or from a vein), how it is obtained (shallow or deep finger stick, alternate site), how the blood is processed (fresh sample, stored or frozen blood), who performs the test (patient user, a lab technician), what reference method is used, and who compares the meter result with the laboratory standard.

Finally, the performance of a meter may not be the same at every glucose value, so it is important that a wide range of glucose values are evaluated and that enough samples are tested in each range. As a consequence, comparing results from two separate studies has a strong possibility of giving an erroneous impression of the comparative performance of two devices.

Even published studies might have misleading conclusions unless they have been carefully constructed to avoid these sources of bias and the reviewers are aware of all of these pitfalls. In other words, it is a very rigorous process to provide a fair comparison. It is also important to remember that the manufacturers are regulated by the FDA with regard to what they may say about any of their products marketed in the U.S. Because of the limitations noted above, the FDA has been cautious about allowing manufacturers to make head-to-head comparisons.

My colleagues at Bayer and I are committed to providing just this kind of quality data. We believe that there are ways to overcome these many technical hurdles to providing the best information to our patients and customers about our products. We are working with advocacy organizations, such as the American Diabetes Association, and regulatory authorities, such as the FDA, to move this process forward.

When to Get a New Blood Glucose Meter?

I have had my current glucose meter for over 10 years. When should one consider getting a new meter? As long as the manufacturer still makes the strips, does it matter? Can meters become unreliable?

K. A., Chattanooga, TN

Belinda Childs, APRN, MN, BC-ADM, CDE, responds: When I am asked this question in the office, I usually answer that the glucose meter you are using is acceptable as long as it is giving you accurate readings. The best way to know if your meter is accurate is to use the glucose control solution for your brand of glucose meter and strips. The meter companies recommend that you do this with each new bottle of test strips and any time you suspect that you may not be getting accurate readings. However, the glucose control solution is generally only good for 30 days after you open the bottle.

Some health-care providers correlate meters with lab readings, but you must remember that there can be as much as a 10–15% variation between a home test and a lab result.

The key to your question, though, is that you have not had a new meter in more than 10 years. Technology has improved significantly over the past decade. Meters now require much less blood, and thus a smaller needle stick. This means less pain and bruising. With many meters, you can also use alternate site testing (on the fleshy part of your palm or forearm as indicated by meters that accept blood samples from alternate sites) and give your fingertips a break. But use your fingers when blood glucose is changing rapidly, such as after a meal, during or after exercise, or when you suspect you have low blood glucose.

Test strip technology is better, too. Some strips allow reapplying blood on the same strip if there's not enough there to get a reading, so you do not use as many strips (and save on cost). Most manufacturers have removed the need to enter a code or change a code key with each new bottle of strips.

Many meters now have data management programs to help you and your health-care provider make sense of the numbers. You can make a note in the meter regarding the timing of the test, such as before or after a meal.

With all these advances, I'd say it's time to shop for a new blood glucose meter. One hint: you may want to check with your health insurance company to see if it has a preferred glucose meter list. Then ask your diabetes educator about different meters' features and decide which one is best for you. *Diabetes Forecast* publishes an annual consumer guide to blood glucose meters and other diabetes supplies. The most recent guide is available at www.diabetesforecast.org/consumerguide.

How Can I Heal Bruised Fingers?

've had type 1 diabetes for over 50 years. For the past 30 years I've used a blood glucose meter, sticking my finger and testing four times a day.

My fingers are starting to turn purple, even though my current meter requires very little blood. Is there anything I can do to heal this?

A. C., San Antonio, TX

Christy Parkin, MSN, RN, CDE, responds:

What to Know: Before testing, wash your hands in warm water and let your arm dangle at your side for a minute or so. This allows the blood to flow down into the fingertips. There is no need to use alcohol if you wash your hands. Alcohol dries and toughens skin over time, making it hard to obtain a drop of blood.

Possible Solutions: To help with bruised fingertips, it may be time to update your lancing device. Newer models are extremely gentle and minimize the trauma of lancing the fingertips several times a day. If you are not using a lancing device already, this will help a lot (some people use the lancet without the device; this definitely hurts more and can cause more bruising). Use the lowest possible setting on the device to avoid a deep stick while giving an adequate amount of blood.

The least painful place to prick is on the sides of the fingertips. Because it is important to rotate sites, be sure to use both sides of the finger. Avoid testing on the pad of the finger; there are more nerve endings there that cause more pain. Pinky fingers can be a great place to prick for the best blood flow.

Some blood glucose meters let you test alternate sites, such as the upper arm, thigh, calf, and palm. These sites contain fewer nerves than the fingertips and may give your fingers some relief. Because there is a lag effect, alternate-site testing should be used only when blood glucose is stable, such as before a meal or when fasting. Always check from your fingertip when blood glucose is changing quickly, such as following a meal, after exercise, or whenever you think your blood glucose might be low.

Although many people reuse their lancets, the lancets will become dull and cause more pain with extended use. Change lancets with each test (or at least daily) to ensure that they are sharp and clean.

Takeaway: Your fingertips may be discolored because of the frequent testing you do, but be sure to discuss this with your health-care provider, as there may be other causes.

Are CGMs Experimental?

My husband has type 1 diabetes. A physician assistant told him the continuous glucose monitor was in the experimental stage (at least in a health insurer's opinion). Is that true?

Name Withheld

Nicholas Argento, MD, responds: No, it's not true! Continuous glucose monitoring (CGM) is now a covered benefit for 70–80% of Americans who have commercial insurance, at least under some circumstances. Unfortunately, though, Medicare and Medicaid do not currently cover home use of CGM.

What to Know: A continuous glucose monitor uses a disposable sensor that is placed under the skin every 3–7 days and sends a signal to a remote receiver. The receiver provides an estimated blood glucose level every 5 minutes. This allows you to track whether blood glucose is moving up or down (and how fast). The receiver can sound an alarm if the level is too high or too low, or if it is rising or falling too rapidly, so you can take action to correct it. This allows you to detect patterns of highs and lows, so that treatments and habits can be modified to safely improve control.

CGM devices do not replace the need for checking blood glucose with a meter, which is used to calibrate the CGM device and to confirm the glucose level if it is going to be used for treatment. There is now a CGM device that will shut off an insulin pump for 2 hours if a low blood glucose level is reached, but only if the person does not clear the alarm.

A landmark study proved that full-time use of a CGM device allows adult patients with type 1 diabetes who have high average blood glucose to lower their blood glucose, with no increase in the risk of hypoglycemia (low blood glucose). A related study proved that a patient with good average blood glucose was more likely to stay in control by using CGM, with less risk of hypoglycemia. Many recent medical studies have reported similar results.

Find Out More: Two companies have CGM devices available in the United States that are approved for use by adults and children: DexCom (www.dexcom .com) and Medtronic Diabetes (www.medtronicdiabetes.com).

Takeaways: CGM is a clinically proven, powerful tool to help people with diabetes who use insulin get their blood glucose under better control and reduce the risk of hypoglycemia. One system will even stop insulin infusion if the person is low and does not respond to the alarm. This lowers the risk of hypoglycemia, especially nighttime hypoglycemia. Most insurance companies will now cover home use of CGM in type 1 diabetes patients and in some people with type 2 diabetes who require insulin, especially those who have problems with hypoglycemia. If insurance refuses to cover CGM, file an appeal. Get your health-care provider's help—ask your provider to send a letter of medical necessity to your insurer.

Why Is A1C Testing Important?

My wife is 78 years old, and she has had type 2 diabetes for many years. Her doctor tells her to get an A1C test every 3 months. Recently, Medicare has denied the claim. Medicare says that A1C is not a covered service and not deemed a medical necessity. I often read about A1C in *Diabetes Forecast*—that it is very important for preventing diabetes complications, such as problems with the kidneys, nerves, and eyes, or cardiovascular events. So, how then can Medicare decide that frequent A1C testing is not a medical necessity? The annual cost for A1C is too expensive ($64.85 per test, four times a year). I might just check A1C twice a year.

C. T., Bayside, NY

Robert A. Gabbay, MD, PhD, responds: You are right that A1C is a very important measure of how a person's diabetes is doing. It is the best indicator and determinant of risk for developing complications of diabetes, as you describe. Since A1C is a measure of average blood glucose for the previous 2–3 months, it gives a good idea of blood glucose control over time. It's important to measure A1C in addition to your regular blood glucose meter tests.

The American Diabetes Association recommends at least two A1C tests a year for patients who are meeting treatment goals and have stable blood glucose. For patients who don't, quarterly A1C tests are appropriate. In most cases, Medicare should cover A1C tests every 3 months for patients with diabetes. But if you get an A1C test as little as a day before the 3-month mark, then it may be deemed unnecessary and Medicare will not cover the cost of the test. Be careful to check this information before scheduling an appointment.

Is My Husband's A1C Too Low?

My husband has type 2 diabetes, and for years his endocrinologist urged him to keep his A1C under 7%. A few months ago we went on a low-carb diet, and my husband lost over 30 pounds. The doctor took him off a sulfonylurea, cut his metformin dose in half, and removed two blood pressure meds.

When my husband's A1C test came back at 6.1%, I thought his doctor would be thrilled. But he said 6.1% was too low. Why?

F. G., Ladera Ranch, CA

M. Sue Kirkman, MD, responds: Although I don't know all the details, I wouldn't necessarily say that your husband's A1C is "too low."

What to Know: The American Diabetes Association recommends that many adults with diabetes strive to keep A1C less than 7%, but the goal can differ from person to person. Even tighter goals, such as less than 6.5%, might be reasonable for people with relatively recently diagnosed diabetes and many years to live. A bit looser goal (such as less than 8%) may be fine for those with advanced diabetes complications, other chronic illnesses, or shorter life expectancies. In all cases, hypoglycemia (blood glucose under 70 mg/dl) should be avoided as much as possible.

Find Out More: The Association's recommendations do not specify a low end of the target range for A1C, because it matters how people get to lower A1Cs. People without prediabetes or diabetes have A1Cs in the mid-5% range or below. Many people with type 2 diabetes can lower their A1C with healthy changes in their diet and exercise, or with bariatric surgery. It would be hard to say that these A1Cs are "too low."

Takeaways: When is someone's A1C considered "too low"? It can be if it's low because of frequent episodes of hypoglycemia, or if it's lower than it needs to be to provide benefit, yet is causing a lot of treatment burden (the expense of multiple medications, for example). It doesn't sound as if that is the case here. Your husband's weight loss and glucose and blood pressure control on fewer medicines are commendable. I hope he'll keep up the good work!

Why Is My A1C Rising?

I am a 36-year-old man who was diagnosed with type 2 diabetes 2 years ago. Until 6 months ago, my A1C was 5.4%, but now it's creeping back to 7%. I am a vegetarian, teetotaler, and non-smoker, and I take oral medication. My diet and lifestyle are unchanged. Why are my blood glucose levels going up? Would eating many small meals help my control?

V. B., Sarasota, FL

Alison B. Evert, MS, RD, CDE, responds: Studies show that the initial treatment of type 2 diabetes with a healthy eating pattern, regular physical activity, and metformin is often successful at achieving optimal blood glucose control. However, type 2 diabetes is a progressive disease. Over time, regardless of which therapies are used, the body's ability to produce insulin declines and more than one type of diabetes medicine may be required.

Blood glucose control is a primary goal of diabetes management, and strategies to reduce blood glucose spikes after meals are important to overall control. The carbohydrate consumed at meals or snacks is the major contributing factor to the rise in postmeal blood glucose levels.

In people without diabetes, the pancreas releases insulin following a meal or snack, keeping blood glucose in a narrow range. In people with type 2 diabetes, though, the inability to release enough insulin, use insulin properly, or both can cause blood glucose levels to become higher than normal. High blood glucose also results both from the overproduction of glucose by the liver and from the amount of carbohydrate consumed.

Nutrition education and counseling can help you determine how much carbohydrate you are eating. You may need to reduce your carbohydrate intake to lower your postmeal blood glucose. If it is found that you are consuming appropriate amounts of carbohydrate, another diabetes medicine may need to be prescribed to improve your control by addressing your body's inability to release enough insulin following a meal.

Your other question about meal and snack frequency is a common one. Nutrition experts have reviewed the research in this area for people without diabetes. Unfortunately, this question has not been studied in people with diabetes. For people without diabetes who are trying to lose weight, several studies show that calories should be distributed throughout the day. It is recommended to eat four or five times per day (meals or snacks), including breakfast. Research has also shown that skipping breakfast is associated with excess body weight and markers of insulin resistance. A word of caution: eating multiple times throughout the day when you're not hungry is likely to result in weight gain and should be discouraged. Again, these findings are for people who don't have diabetes and may not apply in your case.

5

Oral Medications & Supplements

Are My Meds Wearing Off?

I am 63 years old and have had type 2 diabetes for 13 years. I take metformin and glipizide. My morning readings have been 150–180 mg/dl the past few weeks, and I cannot get them down. Is the effect of these drugs going away?

Name Withheld

Belinda Childs, APRN, MN, BC-ADM, CDE, responds: Type 2 diabetes is a progressive disease, and over time, the body is less able to produce insulin. As your body's needs change, additional treatments may be needed.

Lifestyle considerations are important, too. Has there been a change in your meal plan, the timing of your meals, or your physical activity? For example, eating later in the evening can cause an increase in fasting blood glucose levels in the morning.

People with type 2 diabetes may eventually need to take insulin to maintain near-normal blood glucose levels. There are also a range of oral and injected medications for type 2.

The two medications you are taking address three abnormalities of type 2 diabetes. Metformin, a biguanide, both reduces the amount of glucose made by the liver and increases the body's response to insulin. Glipizide, a sulfonylurea, increases the release of insulin from the cells in the pancreas that produce it.

Scientists have learned that other health problems, besides insulin resistance and insulin deficiency, contribute to high blood glucose levels. A number of medications treat these health problems, including thiazolidinediones (TZDs), incretin mimetics, and DPP-4 inhibitors. Pioglitazone (Actos) is a TZD that improves insulin resistance, especially in fat cells. It can be used with metformin and glipizide.

Medications known as α-glucosidase inhibitors delay the absorption of carbohydrate, lowering blood glucose. These drugs (acarbose and miglitol) aren't often used in the United States.

Incretin mimetics lower blood glucose by increasing the insulin release from the pancreas and also by preventing the body from releasing glucagon (which raises blood glucose). They slow the stomach's emptying after eating, too, which may help one feel full sooner and eat less. These medications, which are given by injection, include exenatide (Byetta) and liraglutide (Victoza).

DPP-4 inhibitors have similar effects, but they are taken in pill form and do not slow stomach emptying. They include sitagliptin (Januvia), saxagliptin (Onglyza), and linagliptin (Tradjenta).

Type 2 diabetes is a complex disease. The good news is that there are now many options for treating it, and discoveries keep adding to the treatments available. You'll want to review all the options with your diabetes-care team.

Can Meds Distort My A1C?

M y blood glucose levels are in the range of 160–190 mg/dl, but my A1C is 5.3%, which seems too low. Could my HIV medications be affecting the A1C results?

Name Withheld

Craig Williams, PharmD, responds: Very few things can interfere with the A1C test to give a falsely high or low value. Fortunately, no commonly used medications, including those for HIV, are known to throw off A1C results.

A1C inaccuracies are rare and usually stem from abnormalities in hemoglobin, the part of a red blood cell that gets "glycated" with glucose to form the A1C in the bloodstream. In certain types of anemia (deficiency or alteration in the function of red blood cells), the interaction between hemoglobin and blood glucose is not normal. The laboratory doing the A1C test can often work out these interferences, however, and so the risk of an inaccurate A1C result being reported to a patient or doctor is very, very low.

There are other reasons why an A1C and average glucose readings may not match up, though. Probably the most common is that a person may test blood glucose at just one time of the day and not get a good picture of his or her 24-hour control. For example, if your blood glucose runs high in the morning, and that is always when you check, then your A1C may seem to be falsely low.

In your case, an A1C of 5.3% seems falsely low for average blood glucose in the range of 160–190 mg/dl. A good way to compare an estimated average glucose (eAG) with an A1C is to plug the measured A1C value into the estimated average glucose calculator at www.professional.diabetes.org/glucosecalculator.aspx. The eAG for an A1C of 5.3% is 105 mg/dl. (A way to do the conversion yourself is to subtract 2 from the A1C value, then multiply by 30. In this case, 5.3 − 2 = 3.3. Multiply 3.3 by 30, and the result is 99 mg/dl, roughly the same.) So, the A1C of 5.3% does seem too low for blood glucose levels of 160–190 mg/dl. It's possible that your blood glucose meter is inaccurate.

The first step for anyone whose A1C and blood glucose tests seem to be way off is to check that the blood glucose strips being used aren't expired and haven't been exposed to light or moisture. Use the control solution for your meter to make sure that the device and strips are working together as they should. If the meter isn't at fault, make sure to test your blood glucose at different times of day. If that doesn't explain the mismatch, then the A1C test should be repeated in several weeks. If the inconsistency persists, ask your health-care provider's office or laboratory to check for possible problems in the A1C test or ask your health-care provider about medical conditions that might lead to a problem with the test interpretation.

Do My Husband's Meds Work against One Another?

My husband is on an insulin pump and taking Byetta injections as well as Januvia and Actos tablets. Are these all designed to work together, or are one or more working against the others?

J. M., Oklahoma City, OK

Craig Williams, PharmD, responds: Questions about combining type 2 diabetes medications are increasingly common because so many options now exist. Chronic medical conditions other than diabetes (like heart failure or kidney disease) often play an important role in deciding what combinations of medications are best for a particular patient. Without knowing more about your husband, I cannot give specific advice, but let's consider the four-drug combination that you asked about.

Januvia and Byetta belong to related classes of medications. These drugs work on one or more hormones in the gut that affect insulin secretion, appetite, and glucose production by the liver. Actos works differently and improves the effects of insulin in different areas of the body. All of these effects potentially complement insulin action, and it is reasonable to combine any of them with insulin. However, I wouldn't say the combination of all three agents plus insulin is common, especially because Januvia and Byetta have somewhat overlapping effects. There may not be much benefit to using Januvia and Byetta together. But certain combinations work well for certain patients.

In its approval of Actos, Januvia, and Byetta, the U.S. Food and Drug Administration said there were not enough data to routinely recommend that any of these drugs be continued in combination with insulin. In fact, in the past, oral medications were used mostly to delay the need to start insulin. Once a patient went on insulin to control his or her diabetes, oral medications were frequently reduced or stopped altogether. Although some providers still favor that strategy, more are now willing to combine therapies because some oral medications, such as metformin, have shown benefits in combination with insulin. This is particularly true in patients who take only a once-daily injection of background (long-acting) insulin.

If this combination appears to be helping your husband safely maintain blood glucose control, then it may be a good choice for him. But insulin plus these three other medications is a lot, and you and your husband should continue to work closely with his provider to ensure that each one is truly needed.

Can I Stop My Diabetes Medications?

I was recently diagnosed with type 2 diabetes. I am taking 10 mg of glipizide and 500 mg of metformin twice a day. My A1C was 12.5%, but I have been feeling better, and I even stopped taking the glipizide every morning. My blood glucose average is now 170 mg/dl. Is that good, or should I continue to take my glipizide every morning?

R. W., Chicago, IL

Craig Williams, PharmD, responds: Unfortunately, the medications that are used to help manage blood glucose in people with diabetes do not fix the underlying causes of the diabetes itself. As a result, the medications generally cannot be stopped without losing the blood glucose control that they were providing.

Lifestyle changes can alter the need for long-term medications though, and sometimes enable people with type 2 diabetes to stop taking them altogether. For those who have lost a substantial amount of weight or have significantly increased their exercise routines, it is not uncommon to be able to reduce the dosages of medications, or even to try stopping medication for a period. Reducing or stopping your medications, however, should always be done under the supervision of your health-care provider.

When we do stop therapies or reduce the dosages that are used, our goals for blood glucose control remain at an A1C of less than 7%, a fasting morning blood glucose below 130 mg/dl, and random and postprandial (after eating) blood glucose levels below 180 mg/dl. If those targets can be maintained with lower doses or no drugs at all, then it may be safe to change your regimen. Because your A1C and average blood glucose are not in those ranges, you probably need to start your medication again to achieve blood glucose control.

Should I Change My Medications because of the "Dawn Phenomenon"?

I have had type 2 diabetes for 2 years and take metformin with dinner. My fasting blood glucose is between 110 mg/dl and 140 mg/dl. My 2-hour postmeal readings, however, are the same, even though the fasting levels should be lower than the 2-hour readings. I seem to have something called the "dawn phenomenon." My doctor agrees but hasn't changed my medication. Is there a different way to treat this so that my fasting readings would be lower?

B. S., Naperville, IL

Roger P. Austin, MS, RPh, CDE, responds: All people experience the "dawn phenomenon," whether or not they have diabetes. The dawn phenomenon is caused by a surge of cortisol and growth hormone that the body produces during the night. The result of this surge is an increase in fasting blood glucose levels that often happens around 4:00 to 5:00 a.m.

The body's normal insulin response adjusts for this, so people without diabetes never notice any change in fasting blood glucose levels. However, people with diabetes do not have normal insulin responses, and therefore they may see an increase in fasting glucose. This is primarily because they are producing less insulin and more glucagon (a hormone that increases blood glucose) than they need. The less insulin produced by the pancreas, the more glucagon the pancreas makes as a result. Glucagon, in turn, signals the liver to break down its storage supplies of glycogen into glucose. This is why high fasting blood glucose levels are commonly seen in patients with type 2 diabetes.

What can be done to correct this? Eating dinner earlier in the evening and engaging in some light physical activity after dinner can help. However, if the fasting glucose continues to be high, this may suggest the need for medications that can help to control the insulin–glucagon relationship. The most commonly used medications are metformin and the once- or twice-daily long-acting insulins, glargine and determir (Lantus and Levemir). Because you already take metformin, you may want to discuss with your health-care provider the need to adjust your dose, or the possible addition of long-acting insulin.

While Fasting, When Do I Take My Meds?

How do I manage diabetes when fasting for a blood test or a colonoscopy? I had to skip my colonoscopy last year because of low blood glucose. And now I have to have a cholesterol test. What do I do?

Name Withheld

Nina Watson, MSN, RN, CDE, responds: Fasting can be a challenge for people with diabetes, especially when you are taking medications that have a direct effect on your blood glucose level. Always discuss how to adjust your medication regimen with your health-care team before the fast. The changes you make will depend on what medications you are taking, the dosages, your blood glucose control, how long your fast will be, and why you are fasting. For instance, someone with diabetes who is having a procedure should request to have it done early in the day to avoid prolonged fasting.

Here are some general rules to follow for a morning fast. If you're on oral medications, hold them until the test is complete and take them when you're ready to eat. If you are taking metformin and the test involves an intravenous injection, you may need to hold the metformin until at least 48 hours after the test (this is to ensure that your kidney function remains normal). Stop any noninsulin injections such as Byetta and Symlin that are only to be taken with meals, and take those when you are ready to eat again.

Insulin changes are dependent on your prescribed regimen. Mealtime insulins, such as NovoLog, Humalog, Apidra, and Regular, should also be held until you are ready to eat. Dosing of background (long-acting) insulin should be discussed with your health-care provider. If you are on Levemir or NPH at bedtime only, there should be no need to hold your injections. If you take long-acting insulin twice daily, your provider may want you to decrease the dose depending on the length of your fast, your blood glucose control, and your risk for hypoglycemia. If you take Lantus, your provider may or may not adjust your dose, based on how much of it you are taking and how long your fast is anticipated to be. If you use an insulin pump, consult with your health-care provider about any needed changes to your basal (background) insulin rate.

No matter what type of diabetes medications you take, check with your doctor for a detailed plan that you can follow when you're scheduled for a procedure that requires fasting. It is always a good idea to plan ahead.

Should I Be Taking Avandamet?

keep seeing warnings about the drug Avandia. I am currently taking Avandamet, a combination of Avandia and metformin. I had a heart attack in 1998 and was diagnosed with diabetes 5 years later. An endocrinologist put me on Avandamet, which I have taken ever since. Should I be concerned?

D. W. R., Elyria, OH

Craig Williams, PharmD, responds: Patients and doctors are still confused about the decisions and changes in decisions that have occurred around the medication rosiglitazone. In 2010, the U.S. Food and Drug Administration (FDA) decided that the benefits of rosiglitazone (Avandia, Avandaryl, and Avandamet) for controlling blood glucose generally did not outweigh an apparent increased risk for heart attacks. That ruling laid the groundwork for a restricted access program that remained in place for about 3 years and severely limited the use of all products containing rosiglitazone. The decision to implement the restriction program in 2010 was controversial and was something that not everyone agreed with. In November 2013, after reviewing a few sources of new information about rosiglitazone, the FDA released a new statement saying that it is reversing its decision about the increased heart attack risk for rosiglitazone and that it will be eliminating the increased restrictions on the prescribing of rosiglitazone. Similar to its cousin, pioglitazone (Actos), rosiglitazone will still have a warning about the possibility of increasing the risk of heart failure, but it will no longer carry a warning about an increased risk of heart attack. As of early 2014, these new changes were still being implemented.

Should I Be Worried about Actos?

I was diagnosed with diabetes 1 year ago and was placed on Actos. I am concerned about continuing on Actos based on all I read about it, and I have not tried any other treatment. Should I be concerned, and would you recommend other treatments?

M. P.

Craig Williams, PharmD, responds: Many readers will be aware of the recent controversy surrounding the "glitazone" drugs, rosiglitazone (Avandia) and pioglitazone (Actos). The controversy began with an analysis that looked back at about 40 mostly smaller studies with rosiglitazone and determined that there was a small but significant increased risk of heart attack with that drug. To put it in some perspective, there was about one extra heart attack for about every 2,000 patients treated for a year with rosiglitazone. So far, similar analyses with pioglitazone have not found the same risk, and a large randomized trial of pioglitazone completed in 2005 actually found a small reduction in the risk of heart attacks. Additionally, in 2013 the FDA decided that the original risk that appeared to be present for rosiglitazone (Avandia) was actually much lower than it appeared, and the warnings about that risk were eliminated in 2014. However, many clinicians and researchers remain aware of the original data and are still skeptical that rosiglitazone is really as safe as other diabetes medications.

There were always some real limitations on the data available for the original analysis that showed the risk with rosiglitazone. Shortly following the original study that showed some risk, a large randomized trial of nearly 4,500 patients taking rosiglitazone for nearly 4 years failed to show an increased risk of heart attack compared to sulfonylureas and metformin. It was partly an independent reanalysis of that prospective study that convinced the FDA in 2013 that rosiglitazone does not carry an increased risk of heart attack. But while the controversy continues, do not forget that the risk of poorly controlled hyperglycemia is quite clear, so no one should stop taking glucose-lowering medications without consulting his or her primary-care provider. Also, there is already a well-known risk with both agents among patients with heart failure. None of the recent controversy has lessened that concern.

So in regard to the specific question of pioglitazone, the data to date have not shown any increased risk of heart attack and it can and should remain a part of a comprehensive diabetes management strategy for appropriate patients.

Does Lantus Cause Cancer?

did a Google search on the side effects of Lantus, and one site I found said Lantus may cause cancer. I have type 1 diabetes and have taken Lantus as my long-acting insulin for about 5 years. It works pretty well, but now I'm starting to worry. A coworker who also takes Lantus may have throat cancer. Could they be connected?

G. V., Roseburg, OR

M. Sue Kirkman, MD, responds: There is no clear evidence that Lantus, or any other insulin or diabetes medication, causes cancer. In the summer of 2009, four research papers about diabetes medications and cancer risk were published in the journal *Diabetologia*. All four studies were from European countries and looked at existing data on large groups of people. Some, but not all, of the studies suggested that people who took Lantus had a higher risk of some forms of cancer, especially breast cancer.

There has been disagreement in the medical and scientific community about the ways the study results from 2009 were analyzed, and whether the findings are "real" or not. As with any observational study, even if a higher risk of cancer was seen in people who take Lantus, that doesn't mean that Lantus caused the cancers. It may be that some other risk factor for cancer was more common in Lantus users than in those who didn't use it. The best way to account for these confounding variables is through a randomized controlled trial, where people are assigned to one treatment or another through a random process that is like flipping a coin. If the study is large, the confounding factors, even if we don't know what they are, should be found in roughly equal proportions in both groups. There have been a number of randomized trials comparing Lantus with other forms of insulin, and none of them have shown higher rates of cancer in people assigned to take Lantus, so this is reassuring.

Independent of Lantus or other diabetes medications, there is evidence that people with diabetes, especially those with type 2 diabetes, may be at higher risk of some forms of cancer, such as colon cancer and breast cancer. The reasons for this are not clear, but possibilities include the links between type 2 diabetes and obesity (itself a risk factor for cancer), high blood glucose levels, or insulin resistance. No studies have suggested any link between throat cancer and diabetes (or Lantus).

In short, I don't think you should be concerned about your therapy, especially if it is working well for you. Like all adults, people with diabetes should get recommended cancer screenings and should try to avoid known risk factors for cancer, such as smoking, obesity, and physical inactivity.

Would a Blood Pressure Medication Help?

M y 28-year-old son has had type 1 diabetes since he was 14. A health-care provider recently prescribed lisinopril, a blood pressure medication, saying it had been shown to help people with diabetes protect their kidneys.

My son's A1Cs are usually in the 7% range, and he is apprehensive about starting on a new medication. Does it help? What are the risks of not taking it?

K. F., Grand Blanc, MI

Roger P. Austin, MS, RPh, CDE, responds: Thank you for asking—protecting the kidneys is an important part of living well with diabetes, and the American Diabetes Association hopes to raise awareness of the issue. Kidney damage (also called nephropathy) occurs in 20–40% of people with diabetes and is the single leading cause of end-stage renal disease (ESRD).

What to Know: Low levels of albumin in the urine have been shown to be the earliest stage of diabetic nephropathy in patients with type 1 diabetes. Persistent albuminuria at modestly elevated levels of 30–299 mg/24 h is also a marker of increased risk for cardiovascular disease (heart attack and/or stroke).

Albuminuria is detected by a simple urine test called the albumin-to-creatinine ratio. This test can show whether small amounts of albumin are present in the urine, indicating that steps are needed to avoid further kidney damage.

Lisinopril belongs to a class of blood pressure medications called angiotensin-converting enzyme inhibitors (ACE inhibitors). ACE inhibitors and the angiotensin-2 receptor blocker (ARB) class of blood pressure medications are especially effective in delaying the progression of diabetic nephropathy, even if the person with albuminuria does not have high blood pressure.

Find Out More: Your son may want to ask his health-care provider if the test for albuminuria has been done and how the provider has interpreted the results. The test is recommended once a year for all people with type 2 diabetes and for people who have lived with type 1 diabetes for 5 years or more. The healthy target is less than 30 mg/24 h.

Takeaway: The combination of blood glucose control (as evidenced by your son's A1C of 7%) and blood pressure control is particularly effective in reducing the progression of diabetic nephropathy.

Why Do I Take an ACE Inhibitor?

I have had type 1 diabetes for 40 years and I am in good health. I've been on the insulin pump for 10 years. My last A1C was 7.8%, which was high for me. Why do I need to take an ACE inhibitor?

I have been taking one for 12 years. I do not have high blood pressure or any heart problems. The side effects for me are dry mouth, skin rash, and headaches, and the medication just doesn't seem to be worth it. Please provide some perspective. While I respect my doctor, I haven't gotten a satisfactory explanation as to why I am taking it.

J. D., Tucker, GA

Roger P. Austin, MS, RPh, CDE, responds: Angiotensin-converting enzyme (ACE) inhibitors are a class of blood pressure–lowering medications that have a wide variety of therapeutic uses. In addition to controlling blood pressure, they are used in a number of heart conditions, including heart failure, coronary disease, and heart attacks. They also are used in cerebrovascular disease, and have particular application in diabetes because of their role in preventing and treating diabetic kidney disease.

Because you don't have high blood pressure or any heart problems, you should discuss the status of your kidney function with your health-care provider. ACE inhibitors are first-line medications in treating albuminuria, which is the leakage of small amounts of protein into the urine. It is one of the first signs that your kidney function may be declining as a result of sustained high blood glucose levels, high blood pressure, or both. ACE inhibitors can be used in response to modestly elevated albuminuria—for people with either type 1 or type 2 diabetes—even if the patient's blood pressure is normal. It has been said that the ACE inhibitors have a "protective effect" on the kidneys because of the way they affect blood flow to and from the kidneys. Like all medications, ACE inhibitors can cause side effects, which you describe in your letter. Since there are many different ACE inhibitors on the market, ask your health-care provider about trying a different one, which may not cause the side effects you describe. Another alternative is to use an angiotensin-2 receptor blocker (ARB), which can be used in patients who may not tolerate ACE inhibitors. ARBs also have protective effects on the kidneys.

Can ARBs Protect Your Kidneys?

I am a 66-year-old woman with type 2 diabetes. My A1C was less than 6% without medication. My albumin level is less than 3.

I had a problem with my ACE inhibitor: a side effect of constant dry coughing. Recently, my blood pressure has been high, so I started taking Norvasc, which brought my blood pressure down below 110/70 mmHg. I have been told Cozaar, an ARB, will protect the kidneys.

Would you explain the mechanism of how ARBs affect the kidneys? Is there an added benefit to being on an ARB even though Norvasc keeps my blood pressure down? If so, what is the optimum dose of Cozaar to protect the kidneys? My cardiologist said a higher dose is better.

E. Y., Shavano Park, TX

Craig Williams, PharmD, responds: Angiotensin receptor blockers (ARBs) and angiotensin-converting enzyme inhibitors (ACE inhibitors) have special effects that protect the kidneys in a way other blood pressure–lowering medicines don't. ARBs and ACE inhibitors achieve this through reducing the effects of the hormone angiotensin 2.

In the kidneys, angiotensin 2 constricts the blood vessels in an especially harmful way, which results in an elevated blood pressure in the kidney that is often more severe than elevations in systemic blood pressure (what we measure with the cuff on the arm). In fact, damage to the blood vessels in the kidney and elevated kidney blood pressure can occur before any elevation in the blood pressure you typically measure. To watch for this early damage, we monitor for protein in the urine (proteinuria). You mentioned that the amount of protein in your urine (your albumin) is normal (anything less than 30 mg/g creatinine or 30 mg/24 h is considered normal). That is very good. The numbers that you describe (blood pressure of 110/70 mmHg and normal albumin excretion) are at their goals.

In general, both the National Kidney Foundation and the American Diabetes Association agree that patients with an elevated blood pressure or abnormal proteinuria should be on an ACE inhibitor or an ARB, with a goal of reducing proteinuria and achieving a blood pressure of less than 140/80 mmHg. Although higher than normal doses of either class of medicine can have a greater effect on lowering proteinuria and may be needed to achieve blood pressure goals, it is not clear if there are benefits to those higher doses if blood pressure and proteinuria are already at goal on standard doses.

In general, ACE inhibitors or ARBs should be used in at least standard doses to achieve blood pressure goals and to lower proteinuria. Side effects to watch for at normal or higher doses are hypotension (low blood pressure), an elevated amount of potassium in the blood, and, as you noted, a dry cough with an ACE inhibitor. A condition called angioedema can occur with an ACE inhibitor and it can also happen with an ARB in patients who experienced it with an ACE inhibitor. Angioedema is characterized by swelling, or edema, around the face and neck.

Despite how good ACE inhibitor and ARB medications sound, not every patient with diabetes should be on one. Although some experts like to debate this point, patients with diabetes who have a normal blood pressure without blood pressure medication and normal albumin excretion can be safely followed without being put on an ACE inhibitor or an ARB. But it is important to have good medical supervision so that therapy can be started if either risk factor appears. Your doctor should check your blood pressure at every visit and screen for proteinuria at least once a year.

Can Statins Cause Pancreatitis?

was diagnosed with type 2 diabetes in 2002. About 5 years ago, I was diagnosed with pancreatitis and was hospitalized. One of my doctors said that the cholesterol-lowering statin Lipitor could have caused the problem since I had none of the other associated problems that can cause pancreatitis. I had been on the lowest dose of Lipitor for only 6 weeks before getting pancreatitis. I know of two other people, both of whom had had their gall bladders removed, who got pancreatitis after taking the statin Zocor.

A few months ago, I had a recurrence of my pancreatitis. I have not taken any statins since going off Lipitor after my first pancreatitis attack. I wonder if taking statins can cause pancreatitis and whether anyone without a gall bladder would be well advised not to take a statin.

G. A., Arvada, CO

Craig Williams, PharmD, responds: There are some case reports of pancreatitis that may be linked to statin use, and the U.S. Food and Drug Administration considers it a possibility, but it is certainly very uncommon. In a large review of 14 placebo-controlled studies of statins, which involved nearly 100,000 patients followed for an average of 5 years, participants on statins had no more instances of pancreatitis than the control group.

You also ask about the possible effect of gallbladder removal on the risk for pancreatitis. Inflammation and irritation of the gallbladder (which is called cholecystitis) is separate from pancreatitis, but they can occur together, and one condition can affect the other, as the pancreas and the gallbladder are connected through the bile duct. I don't know of any reason why someone who has had his or her gallbladder removed should be at a higher or lower risk for pancreatitis.

Although cholecystitis is not listed as a possible side effect of statin therapy, most drugs that are significantly metabolized by the liver (like statins) get excreted partly through the bile. So it's possible that cases of cholecystitis and pancreatitis could occur when using medications that pass through the liver. Yet cholecystitis and pancreatitis also occur in people who are not on any medications, so the occurrence of either one while taking a particular drug doesn't necessarily imply a cause-and-effect relationship.

The best indicator of a drug reaction is improvement of symptoms after a patient stops taking the drug and recurrence of symptoms when the drug is being taken again. Each person responds individually to medications, though, and problems should be handled on a case-by-case basis with your health-care provider.

Does Cinnamon Conflict with Metformin?

I've heard that cinnamon helps control blood glucose. How much truth is there to this, and would it in any way conflict with my taking metformin?

T. C., Claremore, OK

Roger P. Austin, MS, RPh, CDE, responds: Cinnamon has been used as a spice and for medicinal purposes for thousands of years. Medicinal uses have varied over the centuries and include a wide variety of maladies such as gastrointestinal disorders, chronic bronchitis, rheumatism and arthritis, and toothaches. More recently, there has been a flurry of interest in the effects of cinnamon on blood glucose levels. A number of scientific papers have looked more closely at these effects, but the conclusions are mixed at best. Some studies showed that cinnamon lowered fasting blood glucose, total cholesterol, and LDL ("bad") cholesterol. Other studies showed no effect on insulin sensitivity, blood glucose levels, or cholesterol. Ultimately, there is insufficient evidence to support the use of herbs and supplements, such as cinnamon, in the treatment of diabetes.

This serves to illustrate one of the classic problems with the widespread interest in "natural" or "herbal" remedies for treating human diseases. First, there are several different sources of cinnamon. Cinnamon can be derived from the bark of several species of cinnamon trees or from their leaves; there are a variety of processes used to extract and to refine these products as well. Cinnamon comes from various countries, and is grown in different climates and at different altitudes, all of which can affect the content of the active compounds. Most natural sources of cinnamon are from Asia, including China, Vietnam, Indonesia, and Sri Lanka. Thus, when one purchases "cinnamon," there is no international standard for the content of active ingredients that may have effects on blood glucose or cholesterol. Furthermore, the U.S. Food and Drug Administration does not regulate the content of active ingredients in any of the many herbal products sold in the United States.

So, could the regular use of cinnamon (other than as a spice or flavoring) conflict with your use of metformin? We have no way of predicting to what degree, if at all, cinnamon affects metformin. In contrast to the lack of regulation of herbal remedies, the FDA does strictly supervise and monitor prescription and over-the-counter medications manufactured and distributed in the United States, for both safety and efficacy. When you take your regular dose of metformin, you can reasonably expect a consistent effect on your blood glucose levels. You do not have the same assurance when you choose to use an unregulated substance such as cinnamon.

Can Steroids Have a Lasting Effect on Blood Glucose?

Three years ago, when I was 65 years old, I was prescribed prednisone during a very bad cold. I have type 2 diabetes, which I controlled then with diet and exercise (no medications). After I started taking prednisone, my blood glucose shot up to 300 mg/dl, and it took me 3 weeks on Actos to bring it back down. My blood glucose has never been the same, and now I am on diabetes meds. Could the prednisone have caused a lasting effect?

R. W., Stormville, NY

Roger P. Austin, MS, RPh, CDE, responds: Prednisone is a commonly prescribed corticosteroid (steroid, for short). These drugs have also been called "glucocorticoids" because of their effects on glucose metabolism: increases in blood glucose are common among people taking prednisone and other steroids. Prednisone is a synthetic steroid that is used to treat a wide variety of inflammatory conditions, such as bursitis and arthritis in the joints. It's also prescribed for its immunosuppressive properties: for allergic reactions, acute flare-ups of asthma, autoimmune conditions, antirejection treatment after transplant surgery, and cancer chemotherapy, among many other uses.

People with diabetes receiving steroid treatment should be informed that their blood glucose will increase while they are on the steroid. Doctors should help patients determine what adjustments are needed to keep blood glucose levels within the target range.

In your case, since you weren't already taking any medication for lowering blood glucose, Actos was prescribed. Actos, a thiazolidinedione, can take as long as 4–6 weeks to have any measurable effect on lowering blood glucose. Treatment with a faster-acting diabetes medication such as insulin, or a sulfonylurea such as glipizide, will control the elevated blood glucose during steroid treatment, and may have worked better for you.

Steroid treatment is usually prescribed for short periods of time, and your blood glucose should return to pretreatment levels a few days after the steroid is stopped. So, it is unlikely that your continued high blood glucose levels are due to the short course of prednisone treatment you had 3 years ago. If you still have high blood glucose, you should discuss other options for long-term control with your health-care provider. Type 2 diabetes is a progressive disease and often one or more medications are needed to control it over time.

Is Glucosamine Safe for Me?

I am 71 years old, and I have type 2 diabetes. Last year I developed joint problems in both shoulders. Doctors have prescribed physical therapy, which has helped some but not very much. The supplement glucosamine has helped several people I know who have similar shoulder problems. However, these people don't have diabetes. I want to try the supplement, but I have read that glucosamine may contribute to insulin resistance.

E. B., Rio Vista, CA

Craig Williams, PharmD, responds: Glucosamine is safe to try but it may not be effective. Although there are anecdotal reports of patients with diabetes experiencing slight elevations in blood glucose with either glucosamine hydrochloride or glucosamine sulfate, in the few human studies that have been carefully done, no effect can be detected. These studies are often based on glycated hemoglobin (hemoglobin with glucose attached to it—not a direct measure of glucose levels), and the studies pool the results from many patients, so it is always possible that some individual patients may experience slight changes in blood glucose. Monitoring would obviously be prudent. But again, we consider it safe to try in patients with diabetes.

However, glucosamine being safe doesn't mean that it's effective. Controlled clinical trials have not found a significant positive effect, but some individual patients do seem to experience a benefit. Glucosamine is important for the repair and maintenance of healthy cartilage in joints, but taking it in an oral form may not get it to where it needs to be in an amount that will do any real good. Much of it is broken down in the stomach and digestive tract. Even short trials where similar compounds are injected directly into arthritic joints have not found a significant benefit, and a large study published in the *New England Journal of Medicine* in 2006 did not find a benefit of orally administered glucosamine plus chondroitin sulfate in patients with painful knee osteoarthritis.

That being said, I have had patients who felt strongly that they benefited from therapy. As long as it is not used in place of physical therapy and appropriate rehabilitation and strengthening exercises, glucosamine may be able to play a role for some patients in helping them to manage their pain. Other agents that we use for pain control have their own side effects, and being able to use less of those medications is often a good outcome all by itself. If you do start glucosamine or chondroitin, make sure to keep your primary healthcare provider in the loop and remember, too, that they are both considered nutritional supplements, not medications, and therefore are not evaluated or regulated by the U.S. Food and Drug Administration.

Should I Try
Chromium Tablets?

I take metformin twice a day and, after breakfast, six or seven supplements I've seen mentioned on TV. Now I've ordered chromium GTF because it's reported to help with blood glucose control. Would you recommend these tablets, especially for those who have heart disease, as I do?

J. T. F., Jacksonville, FL

Roger P. Austin, MS, RPh, CDE, responds: Chromium is an essential trace element that is associated with carbohydrate and lipid (fat) metabolism. Chromium is sometimes referred to as "glucose tolerance factor" (GTF), but GTF is actually a complex of various compounds, of which chromium is thought to be the active component.

Some evidence shows that taking chromium picolinate can decrease blood glucose, insulin levels, and A1C and increase insulin sensitivity in people with type 2 diabetes. But not all the evidence is positive, and some studies have been inconclusive because of their small size or other factors.

There is wide interest among people with diabetes about the role of various dietary supplements, herbs, and other "natural" products that may influence blood glucose levels and glucose control. However, use of such products is largely a case of "buyer beware." This is primarily a result of a law enacted in 1994 called the Dietary Supplement Health and Education Act (DSHEA). David Kessler, a former commissioner of the U.S. Food and Drug Administration (FDA), has said that DSHEA "does not require that dietary supplements be shown [by manufacturers] to be safe or effective before they are marketed. The FDA does not scrutinize a dietary supplement before it enters the marketplace."[1] In other words, the law lets manufacturers market herbal products without having proved their safety and efficacy. The FDA can only remove such products from the market later if problems happen to be detected.

Contrast this with the strict standards by which the FDA scrutinizes any new prescription medication before deciding whether to approve its use in humans. New drugs must be proved both safe and effective in stringent, randomized controlled trials. In such cases, the burden of proof falls on the manufacturer of the new prescription medication. Even with such strict guidelines, some new medications enter the market only to be withdrawn when used on a wider scale than during clinical trials.

There are no such requirements, scrutiny, or protections with dietary supplements such as chromium. Furthermore, there are no regulations ensuring uniformity and purity of active-ingredient content, consistency

---

1 Kessler DA. Cancer and herbs. *N Engl J Med*. 2000 Jun;342(23):1742–1743.

of labeling, or inspection of processing and production facilities. Thus, people who choose to use such products do so at their own risk. Discuss any nutritional supplements you take (or are considering taking) with your health-care provider.

Can Omega-3 Supplements Trigger Diabetes?

What is your opinion about taking a liquid omega-3 fish oil supplement? My husband started taking one and loves it, but last year his blood tests showed that he might be on the verge of developing diabetes. I was wondering if he should stop taking fish oil, and if it could have caused the problem?

Name Withheld

Christy Parkin, MSN, RN, CDE, responds: There is no evidence that taking fish oil supplements leads to diabetes; in fact, numerous studies demonstrate the valuable benefits of omega-3 fatty acids, which are substances that the body needs but cannot produce on its own.

Current health recommendations include eating omega-3-rich fatty fish two times a week. Another source of omega-3s is fish oil, which is extracted from cold-water fish such as salmon, mackerel, herring, and cod. One benefit of fish oil is improved cardiovascular health. Its potent anti-inflammatory properties may not only help the heart but also ease symptoms of rheumatoid arthritis, Crohn's disease, and inflammatory bowel disease. In addition, fish oil is used to treat depression, bipolar disorder, postpartum depression, anxiety, and schizophrenia. The Alzheimer's Association recommends eating fish to protect against dementia.

So far, scientific evidence suggests that there are no significant long-term negative effects of fish oil in people with diabetes, including no changes in A1C levels, according to a Mayo Clinic report. However, some precautions should be taken when it comes to fish oil supplements. You should buy a pharmaceutical-grade, purified supplement to help guard against potentially harmful contaminants found in some species of fish—though most problems with contaminants tend to arise when eating fish, not when taking supplements.

Other risks apply to specific groups of people. Young children and pregnant or nursing women should avoid the heavy metals that are found in some fish. High doses of omega-3 fatty acids may also increase the risk for bleeding.

Fish oil supplements often cause gastrointestinal upset, and diarrhea may occur, especially with very high doses. The supplements can also have a fishy aftertaste and increase burping, acid reflux, heartburn, and indigestion. You can minimize these side effects by taking the supplement with meals and starting with smaller doses.

According to the U.S. Food and Drug Administration, most people can safely consume up to 3 grams (3,000 mg) per day of omega-3 fatty acids. Young children, pregnant and nursing women, people who are at risk for bleeding, and those who have high levels of LDL ("bad") cholesterol may need to limit their intake of omega-3s in consultation with their doctor or dietitian.

Using Insulin

6

How Does Insulin Work?

How does insulin actually get from the injection site to the bloodstream? When an insulin peaks in 4–6 hours, does that mean it takes that long for the insulin to get into the blood, or does it get to the blood sooner and just get activated in 4–6 hours? What makes one insulin peak in 1 hour and another in 4–6 hours?

C. C., Avon Lake, OH

Roger P. Austin, MS, RPh, CDE, responds: When you inject insulin under the skin, you are actually injecting molecules of insulin, which break apart once injected.

The basic insulin molecule is called a "hexamer," a six-part crystal, which first breaks into groups of two-part molecules called "dimers," which then further break apart into single molecules called "monomers." It is the monomer that is then absorbed into the capillaries and distributed throughout the bloodstream to actually begin lowering blood glucose levels.

The rate at which the insulin molecule breaks down is determined by the arrangement of amino acids in the molecule. The amino acids are assembled in two interwoven chains of a precise sequence. The newer insulins such as lispro, aspart, glulisine, detemir, and glargine each have unique amino acid sequences that in turn control the rate at which the insulin molecule breaks apart. The first three, which are usually used at mealtime, break apart and are absorbed more quickly than Regular insulin. Detemir and glargine, on the other hand, have been altered so that they are absorbed into the bloodstream in a slow and steady manner. (In the past, we had to add different substances, such as protamine and zinc, to prolong the speed at which the insulin breaks apart in the body.)

When we talk about an insulin having its "peak effect," or "peaking," that refers to the time after injection when the dose has its maximum effect. For example, rapid-acting insulins such as lispro, aspart, or glulisine start working within 10–15 minutes after injection, but have their "peak," or maximum effect, usually about 1–2 hours after injection. After that, the action tends to diminish over time, so that the duration of effect from injection to clearance from the body is usually 4–5 hours.

Do I Need Insulin?

My blood glucose readings at bedtime are good, but in the mornings they're high. I have type 2 diabetes and have been on metformin for about 15 years. I am 78 and do a lot of walking and exercise. Is it time for me to go on insulin?

C. C., Enosburg Falls, VT

Janis McWilliams, RN, MSN, CDE, BC-ADM, responds: The decision about whether you should start insulin therapy is best made between you and your health-care provider. However, let's review some information to take into account.

What to Know: The American Diabetes Association recommends general goals of 70–130 mg/dl for fasting glucose, less than 180 mg/dl after meals, and an A1C of less than 7% (for most people). However, new guidelines for those aged 65 years and older were issued in 2013, and they relaxed the A1C goal to less than 7.5% for healthy older adults with diabetes. What is most important, though, is what your provider recommends for you. Your glucose goals can vary based on factors such as your age and medical history. Setting safe glucose ranges is an important part of your medical visit.

It's not unusual to have your highest glucose of the day in the morning. One possible explanation for high morning blood glucose levels is called the dawn effect (or phenomenon), thought to be caused by the nighttime rise in hormones and the subsequent early-morning blood glucose increase that the body with diabetes can't control with its own insulin.

Find Out More: To help your provider determine the cause of your morning highs, check your glucose before you go to bed and once during the night, at about 3 a.m., over a few days to see if there is a pattern. Also, ask your provider whether you are still a good candidate for metformin. Because metformin is excreted by the kidneys and our kidney function decreases as we age, it is not always a good choice for someone up in years or for someone younger whose kidney function has declined.

Possible Solutions: Type 2 diabetes is a progressive disease, and its treatment may change over time. It's wonderful that you walk and exercise. This often helps lower glucose, not only right after the activity but even into the next day. It is possible that another oral medication may help or, as you suggest, a bedtime dose of long-acting insulin may be the best choice.

Takeaway: Many people resist starting insulin but, once they've started, wonder what they were so worried about. Today's fine, short needles make injection easier than ever.

What's behind a Switch to Insulin?

ow do health-care providers decide when it is time to place their patients with type 2 diabetes on insulin?

S. B., Soldotna, AK

Belinda Childs, APRN, MN, BC-ADM, CDE, responds: When you are not reaching the blood glucose goals that you have set with your diabetes-care provider, then a change in treatment is needed. For most people with diabetes, the A1C goal is less than 7%. The goal for fasting blood glucose is generally 70–130 mg/dl, and after meals, blood glucose levels should be less than 180 mg/dl. If oral medications are no longer working to help keep your blood glucose levels within the target range, then it may be time to go on insulin. Sometimes, other options like Byetta or Victoza (both incretin mimetics that are injected) may be used before going on insulin.

Even with the new classes of oral medications and injectables, most people with type 2 diabetes will need insulin at some point. Some patients may start on nighttime insulin to control fasting blood glucose and then add insulin before eating to control the postmeal blood glucose levels.

It is difficult to predict how long someone can use oral medications alone to manage blood glucose. When type 2 diabetes is diagnosed, elevated blood glucose levels are a result of insulin resistance and insulin deficiency. That is, the insulin being made by the body isn't being used properly (resistance), nor is there enough insulin being made to control the blood glucose (deficiency). Diabetes is a progressive disease; by the time you're diagnosed, your body makes only 20–50% of the amount of insulin it should and production can decrease over time. The longer you have diabetes, the more likely it is that you will need to go on insulin. Controlling your blood glucose is what is most important. Whether you take insulin or not, it is a matter of finding the right combination of healthy food choices, exercise (which helps our bodies use insulin better), and medication to safely reach glucose control targets.

Can I Switch to Insulin?

I want to switch to insulin, but my doctor says there is no dose small enough for me.

I was diagnosed with type 2 diabetes in 2000. I have been on oral meds, including glyburide, since the end of the first year. My A1C is below 6%. I do get lows with my orals, usually when I wake up in the morning. My highs tend to be under 200 mg/dl.

I find it hard to believe I have to let my diabetes get worse in order to get the medication that would be best for my body. Is it true that there is not an insulin dose low enough for me?

C. Q., Cayuga, NY

Craig Williams, PharmD, responds: If you are achieving good glucose control with a sulfonylurea (such as glyburide), there would be no benefit to switching to insulin. Although there is a long-standing school of thought that we should be using insulin earlier in patients with type 2 diabetes, there is no evidence for or against this approach if oral medications are working well. Several years ago, some concerns were raised about some of classes of oral medications, which helped to make the case for earlier insulin. However, much of that concern has lessened as we have gained more experience with these medications and studied them in more clinical trials. So, while in 2009 the American Diabetes Association endorsed only metformin, sulfonylureas, and insulin as the most appropriate therapies for managing diabetes, in 2012 the Association said that the list should be expanded to include other medication classes that are equally acceptable. Health-care providers should take the characteristics of the patient (patient resources and support, ability to manage and cope with hypoglycemia, attitudes and expectations about drug therapy) into consideration when choosing an appropriate individual drug regimen.

So, although insulin is tried and true, there are no clear data to show that insulin offers any extra protection or benefit compared with several other doctor-recommended oral medications like glyburide. As long as the same degree of control is safely achieved, a sulfonylurea works fine.

Although insulin is a great drug for many patients, it can have problems of its own (chiefly, hypoglycemia, or low blood glucose), and you shouldn't feel as if you are missing out if you achieve good glucose control with another recommended oral medication. If the metformin and sulfonylureas don't work, other medications should be added to achieve glycemic control. The risk of poorly controlled blood glucose outweighs concerns about newer therapies.

Your blood glucose is already well controlled, and insulin may result in even more hypoglycemia for the same level of control. Therefore, I agree here that with an A1C of less than 6% and some occasional hypoglycemia already, there is no reason for you to switch to insulin, even with an occasional high blood glucose level at or above 180 mg/dl.

What's the Maximum Amount of Insulin to Take?

I am taking Humalog and Lantus insulins: 40 units of Lantus and 85–90 units of Humalog each day. My morning blood glucose is in the 180–200 mg/dl range. I have had several bad bouts of hypoglycemia and am scared that they could occur while I sleep. Is there a maximum amount of insulin I should take? Should I take an additional dose of Humalog at bedtime? Would different brands of insulin be more effective?

R. W., Phoenix, AZ

Christy Parkin, MSN, RN, CDE, responds: The most important concern is the hypoglycemia, or low blood glucose, you are experiencing. Pay attention to when and under what circumstances you have low blood glucose. Is this happening before meals, after exercise, or when you miss or delay a meal? I would suggest that you do a couple of blood glucose tests between 2:00 and 3:00 a.m. to see what is happening during the night. I'd also suggest that you test at bedtime and keep a written log of all episodes of hypoglycemia, with details regarding the time and what events preceded the low blood glucose. This is important information to share with your doctor or other health-care provider in case medication adjustments are needed.

It is possible that the ratio of your Lantus and Humalog insulins is out of balance. As a general rule of thumb, the long-acting insulin (Lantus) should be about 50% of your total daily insulin, and the mealtime insulin (Humalog) should make up the other 50%, and be split among your three meals. Lantus, your long-acting basal insulin, may need to be increased slowly to bring your morning blood glucose down. This may result in your needing less Humalog before meals, which could decrease the frequency of your lows. I do not recommend that you take an additional dose of Humalog at bedtime, as this will actually increase your chances of hypoglycemia during the night.

There is no maximum amount of insulin that one can take. Some people who are very sensitive to insulin may require small doses, and others who are very insulin resistant will require large doses. You need to take whatever amount is necessary to keep your blood glucose in the normal range most of the time without severe hypoglycemia. There is no need to switch to different brands of insulin. It is more important to adjust the insulin doses to minimize your hypoglycemia and to lower your fasting blood glucose. I urge you to address all of these issues with your health-care provider before making any changes.

Can I Change Insulins?

I n 2005, I was put on insulin glargine (Lantus), switching from NPH and Regular insulins. I've had diabetes for 20-plus years. The cost of the insulin keeps going up and, when I reach the Medicare Part D "doughnut hole," is almost $300 a month. My doctor is reluctant to put me back on NPH and Regular insulins or try 70/30 insulin. Would it be difficult to switch?

Name Withheld

Craig Williams, PharmD, responds: Insulin remains our most effective therapy for lowering blood glucose. But using it effectively and safely requires ongoing attention and adjustments from both providers and patients.

What to Know: First, key differences exist in the time over which various insulins will act, and so we cannot just convert unit for unit between different products. Lantus is long-acting and generally effective for about 24 hours after an injection. A combination of two insulin types, 70/30 is 70% NPH insulin, which is medium-acting (about 12–16 hours), and 30% R insulin (Regular), which is short-acting (about 4–6 hours). Second, the action of insulins differs from person to person because bodies differ in how they absorb the medication. So, general rules about converting might need to be adjusted for each individual. Finally, longer-acting insulins have a lower risk of hypoglycemia (low blood glucose) because the amount of insulin in the blood at any one time tends to be lower compared with similar amounts of shorter-acting preparations. It's very important to avoid hypoglycemia.

Possible Solutions: When first converting from a long-acting, once-daily insulin such as Lantus to a regimen with NPH, the total daily dose may need to be decreased by about 20% to reduce the risk of hypoglycemia. The addition of a short-acting insulin such as Regular should be individualized based on blood glucose readings after meals.

Takeaways: Insulin is an effective, highly individualized therapy; patients and providers should feel comfortable in trying—together—different regimens to find what works best. Long-acting, once-daily insulin has a lower risk of hypoglycemia, but it's also fair to consider the costs of insulin in figuring out what is best for you.

Why Do Insulin Needs Change?

W hen I was diagnosed with type 1 diabetes, I started with 22 units of Levemir—dropping down to 7 units. I was told I was in the "honeymoon phase." Sure enough, my units gradually climbed. However, almost 3 years after diagnosis, my insulin needs continue to go up and down. Is this fluctuation common? What can cause it?

B. M., Spartanburg, SC

Christy Parkin, MSN, RN, CDE, responds: Your insulin fluctuations are very common and can be caused by a variety of factors. When you are newly diagnosed, it takes time to figure out all the variables that will influence your daily insulin dose, including insulin-to-carbohydrate ratios, correction factors, basal (background) insulin, the timing of injections, your level of physical activity, and how much insulin you need for the carbohydrate you eat.

As you note, during the "honeymoon phase" of type 1 diabetes, newly diagnosed people may need less insulin at first because the pancreas still produces some insulin. But like other honeymoons, the diabetes honeymoon doesn't last forever. Its length varies (weeks, months, or occasionally up to a year or more), and not everyone has one.

The honeymoon does not mean your diabetes is improving or in remission. When insulin is injected, the pancreas may get a small break from having to produce insulin. This rest period can stimulate the remaining β-cells to begin producing insulin. These cells, however, will also eventually be destroyed by the autoimmune response that characterizes type 1 diabetes, the pancreas will stop producing insulin, and then the honeymoon is over.

After the honeymoon phase, even if you take insulin and "match" it to the carbohydrate grams you eat, the level of glucose in your blood can change unpredictably. Various factors can be at work. The use of certain medications may require changes in your insulin dose to keep blood glucose on target (for example, the corticosteroid prednisone usually requires increasing your insulin dose). During a cold or other illness, your body typically produces hormones that raise your blood glucose. Alcohol can cause either high or low blood glucose, depending on how much you drink, whether you eat food with it or not, and your activity level. Prolonged stress may cause your body to produce hormones that can prevent insulin from working properly.

In women, as hormone levels fluctuate during the menstrual cycle, so can blood glucose levels, particularly in the week before a period. Pregnancy and menopause may also trigger fluctuations in blood glucose.

In short, if your need for insulin is a moving target, that's a troubling but common part of living with diabetes. Your best tools for dealing with it are carefully tracking your food, exercise, and medications; reviewing the results with your diabetes-care team; and making adjustments in lifestyle and medication as you go.

Can I Switch to Once-a-Day Insulin?

| have been injecting 15 units of Humulin N (human NPH) insulin when I first get up and again at 4:00 p.m. each day for years, as directed by my doctor. I carefully regulate my eating, and my A1C is good. Could I change to a once-a-day insulin pen and get the same results?

F. E., Little Rock, AR

Belinda Childs, APRN, MN, BC-ADM, CDE, responds: First, congratulations on maintaining a good A1C on twice-daily NPH. This tells me you have worked hard to be consistent with your meal plan, exercise schedule, and the timing of your insulin doses.

What to Know: NPH is an intermediate-acting insulin. It begins working after 2 hours, has its most potent action (or peak) between 5 and 9 hours, and lasts up to 12–14 hours after being injected. It can last longer in some people, and the action increases with dose size. Insulin glargine (Lantus) and insulin detemir (Levemir) are the only insulins that generally last 24 hours. They are usually peakless and do come in a pen. These insulins will cost more than your Humulin N.

Find Out More: You did not note if you were experiencing hypoglycemia (low blood glucose). Your current dosing schedule could lead to an overlap of doses that could increase your risk of hypoglycemia in the late evening or early night. In addition, because NPH has a peak action, you may actually be covering your meals with the peaks of this insulin if you are eating a late-morning meal and a late-evening meal. If you change to Lantus or Levemir, which have no peaks, you may find that you need mealtime insulin.

The best way to find out how well your current regimen is working is to test your blood glucose levels at different times of day for a few days, until patterns become clear. I'd suggest testing your blood glucose at fasting, before and 2 hours after the start of your meals, at bedtime, and occasionally at 1:00 to 2:00 a.m. The goal for fasting, before-meal, and nighttime blood glucose levels is 70–130 mg/dl; after meals, the goal is under 180 mg/dl. Testing at night will help confirm that you are not going low then. Share the results with your health-care provider.

Takeaways: It is important to verify that hypoglycemia is not occurring with your current insulin and two daily injections. If you and your health-care provider decide to convert to Lantus or Levemir, which provide steady background insulin, it will be important to test after meals to confirm that you do not need mealtime insulin to prevent high blood glucose (hyperglycemia) after you eat.

Should I Worry about Weight Gain with Insulin?

I am almost 20 years old, have had type 1 diabetes for 8 years, and use insulin glargine (Lantus). Should I try to lower the need for insulin to prevent weight gain? I haven't been gaining weight, but I am concerned that I'll get into a cycle of increased insulin dosages and weight gain.

E. P., North Kingstown, RI

Belinda Childs, APRN, MN, BC-ADM, CDE, responds: Insulin has often been given a bad rap for causing weight gain. Generally, if you are taking the right amount of insulin and avoiding excess calories, you will not gain weight. But doing this can be a very difficult balancing act, especially with type 1 diabetes.

What to Know: For blood glucose control, taking the appropriate amount of insulin to cover your meals and snacks while accounting for your level of physical activity is important. The calories you consume include those you eat and drink in meals and snacks as well as calories you take in to prevent and treat hypoglycemia (low blood glucose).

It can seem as if the insulin is causing weight gain. The truth is: too many calories are causing the weight gain, not the insulin. If you are eating more calories than your body is burning and you are taking insulin to keep your blood glucose levels in the normal range, you may gain weight. Taking too much insulin and then having to eat more calories to prevent lows also may cause weight gain.

Find Out More: A consultation with a dietitian can help you determine how many calories you need to maintain your body weight or to gain or lose weight, if that is a personal goal. If you are having frequent lows, especially during the night or while fasting, then you may need a lower dose of long-acting insulin. Lows within 2–3 hours of eating or during or after exercise may require other insulin adjustments. For a week, test your blood glucose levels while fasting, 2 hours after the start of meals, and at 2:00 or 3:00 a.m. Record your insulin doses, and note how much food and caloric beverages you consume.

Possible Solution: These detailed records will help you and your health-care provider see if you are taking the right amount of insulin, as well as allow the dietitian to evaluate your average daily calorie intake. This is the best way to strike the right balance.

Should I Switch Insulin to Lose Weight?

Have any studies been done, other than by Novo Nordisk, to prove that taking Levemir causes little if no weight gain? I have gained a lot of weight taking Lantus, and I don't know if it would be better to switch to Levemir.

L. S., New Milford, NJ

Roger P. Austin, MS, RPh, CDE, responds: Insulin detemir (Levemir) and insulin glargine (Lantus) are both long-acting insulins. There have been a number of published studies comparing insulin detemir with other diabetes treatments. These studies were primarily funded by Novo Nordisk, the manufacturer of insulin detemir. Studies in patients with both type 1 and type 2 diabetes have shown a slight weight loss or slightly less weight gain in patients on Levemir when compared to other treatment options. However, these differences were small, and whether or not some insulins are worse offenders in causing weight gain is unknown owing to a lack of quality data. You may find it useful to discuss a change of insulins with your health-care provider to see what is appropriate in your case; however, in most cases, a significant lowering of A1C will likely result in some weight gain.

Weight gain with insulin use is not necessarily inevitable. The science of developing newer insulins has over time been directed at trying to better mimic the action of naturally produced insulin in the pancreas. The fewer insulin injections given per day, the less the insulin's performance will be similar to that of naturally produced insulin in the body. Understanding appropriate blood glucose targets before and after meals, as well as frequent and regular monitoring of blood glucose, is essential to successful individualization of insulin dosing and weight management. Minimizing weight gain also requires a good understanding of carb counting, practice of portion control, and the counsel of a registered dietitian.

Without oversimplifying, the challenge is to match your dose of insulin as closely as possible to your body's insulin needs throughout the day. This is affected by a number of different factors, including food consumed (especially carbohydrate), exercise, stress, insulin resistance, and more. Weight gain is more likely for people who eat more calories than their bodies burn or those with frequent low blood glucose who must take in more carbohydrate to regulate blood glucose. Additionally, insulin use affects the brain's perception of hunger and satiety, thus affecting appetite and cravings. You should also recognize the influence that other medications you are taking may have on your weight.

Can Insulin Go Back in the Fridge?

After removing insulin glargine (Lantus) from the refrigerator for use, can it be refrigerated over and over again after having warmed to room temperature, or does this degrade it?

Name Withheld

Roger P. Austin, MS, RPh, CDE, responds: For you to get consistent, predictable results when using insulin, carefully follow the insulin manufacturer's recommended storage conditions.

What to Know: Each vial of insulin or box of insulin pens comes with instructions about how to properly store that particular product. Be sure to read and follow these recommendations. As long as vials or pens are stored unopened in the refrigerator (at 36–46°F), they are good until the expiration date on the container. Questions about the insulin's potency start when you open the vial or pen and begin to use it.

Find Out More: Opened vials of the following insulins and mixtures are stable for 28 days either at room temperature (defined by some manufacturers as 77–86°F) or in a refrigerator (36–46°F): insulin glargine (Lantus), insulin glulisine (Apidra), insulin aspart (NovoLog), insulin lispro (Humalog), Novolin N, Humulin N, Novolin R, Humulin R, and mixtures of insulin (Novolin 70/30, Humulin 70/30, NovoLog Mix 70/30, Humalog Mix 75/25, and Humalog Mix 50/50). Opened vials of insulin detemir (Levemir) are stable for up to 42 days at the recommended conditions. Insulin should not be allowed to freeze; if vials or pens are found to be frozen or if the insulin looks like it has particles in it, these products should be discarded and replaced with fresh supplies.

Takeaways: Shuttling opened insulin vials between refrigeration and room temperature does not appear to affect the insulin's potency under these conditions and time periods. However, manufacturers of insulin pens do not recommend storage in a refrigerator once a pen is opened and in use.

Protect insulin from exposure to light and extremes of temperature above and below those noted. Insulin should never be stored in a vehicle, or on windowsills or ledges, where it can be exposed to such conditions.

When traveling, keep insulin on your person or in your carry-on bag. Insulin placed in suitcases that are transported in cargo holds of aircrafts, boats, and buses or in car trunks may be exposed to damaging temperature extremes.

Can I Freeze Insulin? Have Injection Methods Changed?

A s someone who's had type 2 diabetes for 20 years, I often wonder about two things we are told about insulin use.

First of all, why are we told to never freeze insulin and never to use insulin that has ice crystals in it? What if the insulin had been frozen, or partially frozen, at one time, but is now fully defrosted? Is it more dangerous to use insulin that might have been frozen at some point, or to do without?

Second, when I first started injecting, I was told to draw back on the syringe to make sure that no blood came back into the barrel. But now, more and more, we see insulin pens, as well as other injectable medications (such as Byetta), that we cannot draw back on. I'd like to know why it supposedly was an important step previously, but no longer is.

S. B., Flushing, NY

Janis McWilliams, RN, MSN, CDE, BC-ADM, responds: Whenever insulin freezes (below 36°F) it forms crystals and clumps. This affects the molecular structure and thereby the effectiveness of the insulin. You shouldn't experience immediate physical harm, but with the loss of insulin potency, your blood glucose would likely go up.

Insulin vials, either opened or unopened, generally last for 1 month when stored at room temperature (check the manufacturer's temperature recommendations). A bottle is considered open after the first insulin syringe punctures the rubber stopper. Normally, the open bottle of insulin is kept at room temperature while unopened vials are kept in the refrigerator. When unopened and refrigerated, the vials are good until the expiration date. Insulin should not be allowed to sit in the sun or be exposed to temperatures greater than 86°F, as this also could affect its potency. Finally, before using insulin, you should always examine the vial. Insulins that are supposed to be clear (all insulins except NPH and the premixed insulins) shouldn't look cloudy. The vial shouldn't have clumps or anything floating in it, and it should not have a frosted appearance. It should not have changed in color or appearance compared with when you first started using it. NPH and premixed insulins should look uniformly cloudy when you mix them, and should also not contain clumps or small particles.

If using a prefilled insulin pen or insulin cartridges with a reusable pen, storage life at room temperature can range from 7 to 28 days depending on type of insulin. Insulin pens or cartridges already in use should be kept at room temperature. Pens or cartridges that have not had the seal punctured should be kept in the refrigerator. Consult the package insert or check with your health-care professional for directions for your specific insulin. Don't forget to also examine the insulin cartridge for changes in color or appearance, as discussed above.

As for your second question, I have been a nurse for 35 years, and you are correct that we once taught our patients to aspirate insulin syringes before injecting the insulin. This was to avoid injecting the insulin into a blood vessel and was, at the time, the practice for giving any injection. However, insulin syringe technology has improved, and needles have become shorter and finer. Since insulin is given subcutaneously (into the skin), there is little chance of hitting anything other than a small capillary with your syringe. If you do have bleeding at your site of injection, it is likely from nicking a capillary. Just put pressure on the site until the bleeding stops. If this happens often, you may want to talk with your diabetes educator about some tips for improving your injection technique and rotating your injection sites.

Does Insulin Lose Its Punch?

I am on the Medtronic MiniMed Paradigm pump, and I've noticed that my insulin is not as effective toward the end of the MiniMed reservoir. I believe this happens in conjunction with the end of the vial of insulin I draw from as well. Is this common?

I use insulin glulisine (Apidra), and I never use a vial that is more than 30 days old. I use approximately 60–70 units per day. I fill the MiniMed reservoir with 210 units when I replace the insulin.

J. D., Franklin, NJ

Belinda Childs, APRN, MN, BC-ADM, CDE, responds: Insulin sometimes does not seem as "potent" near the end of a pump reservoir, or even near the end of a vial. The U.S. Food and Drug Administration has approved the use of insulin that is in a reservoir for up to 6 days, depending on the brand of insulin.

The studies that determined this time frame were based on how insulin worked in a controlled setting. Insulin's effectiveness in the day-to-day life of the average person with diabetes certainly varies from the lab result, though, and it varies even more from individual to individual. This is part of what makes diabetes so complicated: everyone is different.

If you are using 210 units every 3 days, you would use a vial of insulin about every 12 days. Sometimes people use insulin from more than one vial, which prolongs the exposure to outside factors. If possible, use insulin out of only one vial: that way, you will use it up in a timely manner.

It also may be helpful to look at how you store insulin. Do you keep it in a cool, dry, dark place? Any insulin you have not begun using should be stored in the refrigerator. Protect insulin and other medications from sun, temperatures higher than 86°F, and humidity. Keeping insulin in a warm, humid bathroom or in a sunny area of the kitchen is not advisable.

Your problem may be due not to your insulin but to your pump site. Look at your pump setup and site-change process. Are you reusing the reservoirs? If so, this may contribute to the insulin's growing ineffectiveness. Does your insulin act differently depending on where your infusion site is? Are you rotating pump sites so that you don't use the same half-dollar-sized areas over and over? Sometimes, as it gets close to time for a needle change, insulin absorption may slow. Living with diabetes often requires the skills of a good detective. You will have to explore these different possibilities and consult with your health-care provider if you cannot find a solution or your problem starts to significantly affect your blood glucose control.

What about Postmeal Insulin?

I s there ever a time when you take insulin after your meals?

Name Withheld

Janis McWilliams, RN, MSN, CDE, BC-ADM, responds: For the most part, rapid-acting insulin is administered before meals. Although it may be tempting to treat random high glucoses with some extra rapid-acting insulin at various times unrelated to meals, you should do this only if so advised by your health-care provider or diabetes educator. The effects of insulin can "stack," and too much insulin can result in hypoglycemia (low blood glucose).

There are exceptions. To explain, it helps first to review the different types of insulin. Long-acting basal (background) insulins ensure that your blood glucose remains controlled in response to various hormonal changes and when you are sleeping. Rapid-acting insulins are faster acting and are taken in bolus doses to cover mealtime increases in blood glucose. The use of a basal-bolus schedule is meant to best mimic the function of a normal pancreas. Long-acting insulin is given only via injections. (With an insulin pump, a continuous infusion of fast-acting insulin provides basal insulin.) Rapid-acting mealtime insulin can be delivered by either an injection or an insulin pump.

Basal insulins include long-acting insulin detemir and insulin glargine. Long-acting insulins are taken at the same time every day, once or twice a day. Intermediate-acting NPH insulin can also be given at bedtime, or in combination with a rapid-acting insulin before meals.

Rapid-acting insulins include insulin lispro, insulin aspart, and insulin glulisine. These are usually given about 15 minutes before the meal. Regular insulin, a short-acting insulin, works best when given about 30 minutes before meals.

That said, special circumstances may dictate that insulin be taken post-meal. For example, parents of toddlers or very young children often do not administer the rapid-acting insulin until they see how much (and how many grams of carbohydrate) the child has eaten. And adults who have problems with delayed food absorption (as in gastroparesis), suppressed appetite, or other issues may delay their insulin injection based on recommendations of their health-care provider.

Am I Injecting Insulin Properly?

s it possible to get hard lumps under the skin when injecting insulin? I have experienced this problem while injecting more than one type of insulin, and I know the lumps are not from using the same injection site over and over again because I always rotate injection sites. But I also noticed when I took my postprandial blood glucose reading that I was up higher than normal. I'm curious as to whether the insulin is getting distributed correctly.

R. K., Baltimore, MD

Belinda Childs, APRN, MN, BC-ADM, CDE, responds: Repeatedly injecting any medication or drug into the same area may result in scarring of the skin and the tissue under the skin. This can happen with insulin. Repeatedly injecting into the same site or near the same site can cause lumps. The lumps or tough skin from repeated injections sometimes are called lipohypertrophy. This type of tissue feels spongy and does not consistently absorb the insulin, which can lead to unexplained high or low blood glucose levels. Rotating your injection sites and avoiding the scarred areas for at least 6 months will help reduce the scar tissue at these overused sites, although some sites may need to be retired. So even though you're rotating your injection sites, you may need to avoid problem areas for a longer time.

You can also get a lump under the skin after an injection when insulin pools. The needle may not have gone deep enough, or you may have been pulling the needle out before the plunger had been pushed to the bottom of the syringe.

Another possibility is that the needle may have clipped a small blood vessel, causing it to bleed and form a little blood blister under the skin. That irritation could prevent the insulin from working as well as it normally would, resulting in a high blood glucose level. If this is happening frequently, you may want to try a little longer needle. Insulin pens and syringe needles come in 4-mm, 5-mm, 8-mm, and even longer lengths.

I have also been asked if air in the syringe might cause lumps. I would not expect air to cause a lump, but if there is air in the syringe, that would mean that you're not getting all the insulin you should be, which would also lead to high blood glucose.

Should I Inject Insulin into a Vein?

I am 20 years old and have type 1 diabetes. When I am off the insulin pump, my blood glucose gets unstable and can take more than 48 hours to go down. Two friends told me that to handle this, they just inject a very small amount of insulin directly into the bloodstream. I know it sounds crazy, but this would save me time and money. Is it safe?

Name Withheld

Christy Parkin, MSN, RN, CDE, responds: The short answer is no, no, no! It's not at all safe. This idea not only sounds crazy—it is dangerous.

What to Know: As you know, insulin is needed to regulate your blood glucose, especially as blood glucose levels begin to rise after you eat. When insulin is produced by the pancreas, it is released in small amounts in response to blood glucose levels over the course of several hours. Injecting insulin just under the skin simulates this response most effectively and safely because the insulin works gradually.

When insulin is injected intravenously, the effect is immediate but very short-lived. Instead of the insulin being gradually absorbed into the circulation from tissue, it is immediately available in the bloodstream. This results in abnormally high insulin levels that can cause a rapid drop in blood glucose levels—hypoglycemia. If left untreated, hypoglycemia may lead to unconsciousness.

The usual delivery of IV insulin is with an insulin drip using Regular insulin. This is administered in a hospital setting with medical support and close monitoring. Because of the high risk for hypoglycemia (and the added risk of unsanitary injections causing infection), it is never advisable to inject insulin into a vein without medical supervision.

Possible Solutions: When your blood glucose is too high, you can use a "correction factor" to give extra rapid-acting insulin in small and calculated doses; ask your provider to help you customize your correction factor(s). Also, if you inject your insulin in the abdomen just under the skin, you will most likely have similar absorption rates from injection to injection and be able to match your insulin dose to the carbohydrate grams you eat. You can also minimize the time you spend off the insulin pump—no more than 1 hour.

Takeaways: The practice of "mainlining" insulin should never be done outside a medical setting. It is a recipe for disaster. You say this would save you time and money. There is no time or cost savings if you have even one emergency room visit for an episode of hypoglycemia.

Do I Need a Longer Insulin Needle?

I have been injecting insulin for 2 years. My question is about needle length. I've used a U-100 31-gauge, 8-mm "short" needle because—well, it should hurt less, right? Because I am slightly obese, should I use the 29-gauge, 12.7-mm needle instead?

S. C., National City, MI

Christy Parkin, MSN, RN, CDE, responds: Your question is a common one. As technology improved and shorter needles became available, it was thought that longer needles were still necessary for those who were overweight. Recent research has shown, however, that shorter needles are very effective in delivering insulin into the tissue just under the skin of both lean and overweight people.

What to Know: In just 25 years, we have gone from using 16-mm-long needles that were much thicker in diameter to 4- to 8-mm needles that are very thin (and practically pain-free). But do shorter needles work as well in people with more body fat? Yes, they do. Recent studies using ultrasound to measure skin thickness at four different sites on the body showed there is minimal variation in skin thickness regardless of a person's age, gender, race, or body mass.

Most people have a skin thickness of less than 2.8 mm, which means that even shorter 4- or 5-mm needles will penetrate the skin and reach the subcutaneous tissue. If insulin is injected with a longer needle (over 8 mm), the chance of injecting into intramuscular tissue is greater. That causes more pain and variation in insulin uptake (and thus in blood glucose levels). The width, or gauge, of a needle has more to do with pain than does the length.

Possible Solutions: No matter which size needle you use, injection technique is important. With shorter needles (4–5 mm), inject at a 90-degree angle with no pinching of the skin. If longer needles are used, pinch up the skin to avoid injecting into intramuscular tissue. Also, hold the needle in the skin for 5–10 seconds after you give the insulin (even longer with higher doses) so the medication doesn't leak from the site. For very lean people, pinching the skin and injecting at an angle are recommended even with shorter needles.

Takeaways: New clinical recommendations support the use of shorter needles. A 4- or 5-mm needle is effective for all body types. The needles are long enough to penetrate the skin into the fat layer but short enough not to reach muscle.

Injections: Is This Bump under the Skin Normal?

I have type 2 diabetes and have just started on insulin injections. My first injection was in my outer thigh. After I injected, there was a nickel-sized raised area under my skin. It wasn't red and didn't cause any pain. I injected at night, and when I got up in the morning, the raised area was gone. Is this normal?

Name Withheld

Roger P. Austin, MS, RPh, CDE, responds:

What to Know: The raised area under the skin indicates that you may have injected the insulin just under the skin instead of into fat tissue. You'll want to review your injection technique in person with your health-care professional. Proper technique helps the insulin dose be absorbed as intended. That ensures the insulin is as effective as possible in lowering your blood glucose level.

Possible Solutions: Learning how and where to inject insulin is best demonstrated by a nurse or other skilled health professional in the office so you can see and repeat the techniques demonstrated, and ask questions. With a few practice shots, most people become injection experts. If you take a large dose, ask your health-care provider about splitting it into two injections to improve the absorption rate.

Takeaways: Pinching up the skin before injecting is important if you are using a needle that is 6 mm or longer, to make sure that you are injecting into fat, not muscle. However, pinching up the skin is not necessary if you are using newer, shorter 4- or 5-mm needles. Shorter needle lengths, such as 4 mm (5/32") and 5 mm (3/16"), are increasingly common and are appropriate for any body size. If you are interested in using 4- or 5-mm needles, you should mention this to your health-care provider and find out if your insurance company will cover these newer needles. The middle front of the upper thigh and the abdomen are commonly recommended injection sites, in part because many people have fat to pinch in these locations. Other injection zones include the buttocks and upper arms, but they may be more difficult for you to reach. Rotating injection sites around the body helps prevent skin irritation and growth or loss of fat tissue.

Does Injected Insulin Hold Fat in the Stomach?

I am 83 years old and have had diabetes for 48 years. I have tried for 7 years to lose weight, and I lose it everywhere except my stomach. I've injected insulin in my stomach for 45 years. Is it true that the insulin I inject holds the fat in my stomach? If so, how can I get rid of the stomach fat without moving the injection site to other parts of my body?

P. G., King City, CA

Janis McWilliams, RN, MSN, CDE, BC-ADM, responds: Congratulations on living well with diabetes for 48 years! No, insulin doesn't cause obesity or "generalized" deposits of abdominal fat. Insulin is absorbed and doesn't stay where it's injected. What you may be describing is called lipohypertrophy or insulin hypertrophy. It is a fatty thickening of the lipid tissue, and these soft, grape-like lumps are sometimes felt more easily than they are seen. The most likely cause is repeated injections into the same spot. Because you have been injecting insulin for a long time, you may have done this without realizing it. Generally, if you avoid using these sites for injection, the hypertrophy may decrease, if not disappear. I have seen some reports of using liposuction to treat hypertrophy, but it is not a common practice.

Another key reason to avoid these areas is that when one injects into these fatty lumps, the insulin's action can be erratic, causing poor blood glucose control. These areas are also less sensitive, and they can become favorite sites as the injection is more comfortable. Sensitivity is less of an issue if you use shorter, finer needles, because they cause little pain when injecting.

It is important to rotate sites when injecting insulin, but you can continue to use your stomach for injections as long as you can avoid these problem areas. You may also rotate to other sites like your buttocks, arms, or legs to give your abdomen a breather. Just be aware that different sites have different rates of insulin absorption and that you should never use a site like your leg if you are planning a walk or other activity using your limbs, because the insulin may work much more rapidly than usual and cause hypoglycemia (low blood glucose). Also, there is some evidence that reusing your own insulin needles can be a risk factor for developing lipohypertrophy, so it's best to use a new needle for each injection.

Finally, it is a good idea for insulin users to periodically schedule a visit with their diabetes educator to review technique and any changes that may have occurred in injection therapy.

Why Do Injections Cause Atrophy?

I am 80 years old and have used insulin for 48 years. For years, I used my thighs as an injection site and noticed that the fat on the inside of my right thigh began to atrophy. I am fairly trim, only 5 pounds over my high school weight.

Now I inject into my "love handles." The atrophy continues to the point that I can see my femoral artery and several large veins. My muscle function is not adversely affected. Why does this happen? What can I do about it?

J. R. R., Dallas, TX

Roger P. Austin, MS, RPh, CDE, responds:

What to Know: Injecting insulin has been associated both with loss of fat tissue and with fat growth. A loss of fat tissue under the skin is known as lipoatrophy or lipodystrophy. In extreme cases, this can cause muscle tissues and bones to be more visible. Some people may be more prone to such fat loss than others. Lipoatrophy is uncommon and can often be a sign of an insulin allergy. You should contact your health-care provider right away to see whether a change in the type of insulin you use is needed.

Growth of fat tissue, or fat hypertrophy, is very common. It may appear as lumps or cyst-like formations under the skin where insulin has been injected. Both fat loss and fat growth may be caused by repeated injections in the same areas.

Takeaways: Growth of fat tissue because of repeated injections can be prevented or reduced by regular rotation of injection sites. The most commonly recommended sites are the middle abdominal area just above the belt line, avoiding an area 2 inches from the belly button, and the upper thigh. Loss of fat tissue may be a sign of an insulin allergy and should be discussed with your care provider as soon as possible.

Can Insulin Pumps Cause Infections?

I was on an insulin pump for about 3 years. I was very careful to shower and clean the area where I was inserting the needle for my insulin pump infusion set. I was doing fine for years and then all of a sudden an area of my body would get red and swell, and I would have to change sites every day. Finally one of the sites got badly infected, and I had to be administered intravenous antibiotics for an hour a day for 2 weeks. I had to have surgery to remove the pocket of infection. My doctor then had to take me off the pump and put me back on insulin shots. We decided it must have been some type of allergic reaction to whatever the infusion set was made of. Have you ever heard of this before, and do you know how to handle the situation?

C. C., Holts Summit, MO

Christy Parkin, MSN, RN, CDE, responds: Allergic reactions at the infusion site can be caused by adhesives, coatings on infusion needles, the metals in needles, or by the insulin itself (which is rare). They are remedied by changing the type of infusion set, adhesives, and needles used.

Although it is possible that you had an allergic reaction (called contact dermatitis), these problems usually occur within a couple of days or weeks after initiating use. In your case, you were on an insulin pump for a number of years, so it is more likely that you experienced an infection caused by "staph" (*Staphylococcus aureus*) bacteria. Infusion site infection is the most common complication associated with insulin pumps. And it is one of the most common causes for discontinuation of insulin pump therapy.

If you have an active infection, the reservoir and infusion set must be removed and discarded and another infusion site used until the infection has cleared. Treatment with oral antibiotics is needed. Also, use of a topical antibiotic cream early in the course of an infection will often slow or prevent its spread.

If you continue to have site infections, you should double-check your technique in cleansing the site and changing the infusion set. If these techniques are correct, you should apply a topical antiseptic to the site prior to inserting the set. If you are prone to site infections, you should perform a triple antibiotic procedure before inserting your infusion set. This requires you to:

1. Wash the area with an antibacterial soap and let dry.
2. Cleanse the area with an antibacterial solution and let dry.
3. Apply an antiseptic and adhesive wipe to the area and let dry.

Skin infections are a potential but preventable risk of insulin pump therapy. The main thing to do is to change your infusion site as indicated and use proper technique in preparing the infusion site. Although problems with insulin pump therapy are occasionally related to the pump itself, the vast majority of problems are related to infusion sites and sets. You should always suspect something is wrong with the infusion site whenever you have unexplained high blood glucose or experience any redness, swelling, or pain at the site. When in doubt, always change the infusion set using sterile technique and good hygiene.

Where Can I Find New Insertion Sites?

I've had type 1 diabetes for 28 years and have used a pump for 14 years. I have trouble finding enough good infusion set insertion sites. I primarily stick to my stomach. What other sites could I use?

W. B., Cary, NC

Christy Parkin, MSN, RN, CDE, responds: After years of pump therapy and/or injections, it can be a challenge to find choice "real estate" that offers good insulin absorption.

What to Know: The abdomen is the preferred site for infusion set sites and injections. It is easy to see and reach, and offers the quickest absorption. Alternative sites tend to absorb insulin more slowly than the abdomen. Here are alternative sites:

- Hips and upper buttocks. Even lean people tend to have some extra padding in these spots. Although there is slower absorption here, these areas are good sites for people with low body fat.
- Outer thighs. Absorption may be increased with activity, such as walking or running. The inner thighs aren't recommended, because when the thighs rub against each other, the site can become irritated and at risk for infection.

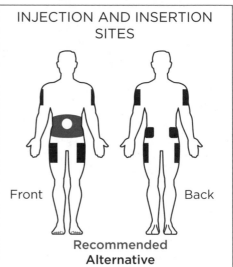

INJECTION AND INSERTION SITES

Front

Back

Recommended

Alternative

- Back of the arms. You may have some extra tissue under the skin here, but the area is hard to reach, especially if two hands are required for insertion. Physical activity can increase the absorption from this location.

Possible Solutions: Inserting too many infusion sets in the same spot over many years can lead to scarring and/or overgrowth of fatty tissue (known as lipohypertrophy), which can cause poor absorption of insulin. Poor absorption may delay the effect of the insulin or require you to use more. If you can feel or suspect damaged tissue under your skin, avoid using the area; it can take several months for the tissue to heal.

Make a plan to regularly use different sites to maintain good skin integrity. Site rotation is a systematic method of selecting various sites so that each one has a chance to fully heal before it is used again. There are several methods of site rotation (see "Site Rotation Patterns"). Choose the method that works best for you.

New sites should be at least 2 inches away from a previous site (as well as 2 inches away from the belly button). Change your site every 2–3 days, depending on the type of cannula you use.

Takeaways: Experiment with some alternative locations to open up your options and keep your sites healthy. And change the infusion set at the first sign of pain, swelling, or redness to avoid tissue damage. Remember, the rule of thumb to live by to preserve your sites is: "When in doubt, change it out."

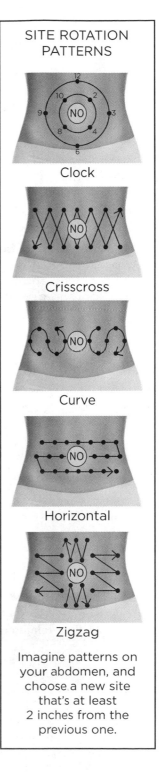

SITE ROTATION PATTERNS

Clock

Crisscross

Curve

Horizontal

Zigzag

Imagine patterns on your abdomen, and choose a new site that's at least 2 inches from the previous one.

Why Won't My Infusion Sets Stick?

I experienced a problem when traveling and hope you can advise me. My infusion sets wouldn't stick. I held the applicator on for the required 20–30 seconds, but when I pulled it off, the set came with it. It sometimes took me three or four tries to get one to work. With the cost, and the fact that I didn't bring more than 5–10 extras along for a month's trip (space is limited on a motorcycle), I became alarmed!

I thought it might be the change in humidity, or the skin-prep wipes. I tried with and without the wipes, so I don't think that was the problem, and I changed my site in the mornings when my skin was cool and dry. Still, I had trouble.

Do you have any idea what might be going on?

S. T., Kamiah, ID

Belinda Childs, APRN, MN, CDE, BC-ADM, responds: One of the challenges of insulin pump therapy can be finding the right site preparation and the right site for the infusion needle.

As with most things with diabetes, everyone is a little different. In my experience, using the skin prep—not alcohol—is important. You might want to try a liquid adhesive like Mastisol if other products do not work.

Site placement may also have contributed to the needle coming out or not holding while you were on the motorcycle. Your arms or hips may be a better choice than your legs or abdomen because of your positioning when sitting on a motorcycle, bike, or similar vehicle. On occasion we have had patients place a wound dressing, such as a Tegaderm dressing, on the skin first, with a hole cut for the needle to go through, and then place the infusion set on top of this dressing. Another alternative is to place the clear dressing over the infusion set to help secure it.

Also let the manufacturer know about any problems you experience with your infusion sets. This way, the company can track any problems and may have suggestions related to that particular infusion set and its adhesive.

Any Tips on Pump Use and Sex?

I am counseling a person who has type 1 diabetes and uses an insulin pump. She is wondering how to manage the pump when she becomes sexually active. Do you have any suggestions?

G. T., MS, LPC, Normal, IL

Janis Roszler, MSFT, RD, LD/N, CDE, FAND, responds: I'm so pleased that you and your patient are having this important conversation! Too many people with diabetes never discuss intimacy with their health-care team. Here are a few tips you can share.

What to Know: People who wear insulin pumps usually have a choice during intimacy—they can disconnect or leave their pump on. If your patient chooses to disconnect, she can safely be away from her pump for about 45 minutes to an hour. But she must remember to reconnect before she falls asleep. Many people find it helpful to set a reminder alarm, as it is very dangerous to go the entire night without any insulin delivery. If she wears a pod-type pump that doesn't disconnect, she should wear her pump on an area of her body that won't interfere with intimate activity.

Possible Solutions: If she leaves her pump on during sexual activity, she shouldn't panic if it gets pulled out accidentally. This is not dangerous. The bleeding that may occur is not harmful. Just have her reconnect when she is done, check her blood glucose level, and treat any abnormal result as directed by you or other members of her health-care team.

Find Out More: To learn how to enjoy a more fulfilling intimate life with diabetes, read *Sex and Diabetes: For Him and For Her*, which I coauthored. It is a fun and informative book that contains personal stories, expert guidance, and even diabetes-friendly recipes that are made with aphrodisiac ingredients. Published by the American Diabetes Association, it is available at www.shop diabetes.org.

Takeaways: Everyone with diabetes can participate in sexual activity. If your intimate life has changed, ask your health-care provider to help you find ways to enjoy it once again.

If I Eat More Carbohydrate, When Should I Bolus?

I use a meter programmed to my insulin pump. After I test for blood glucose and bolus for what I intend to eat, if I am still hungry and want to eat more 10–15 minutes later, can I just bolus for the extra carbs?

Name Withheld

Alison B. Evert, MS, RD, CDE, responds: Yes, if you eat more carbohydrate, you should deliver an additional insulin bolus for this food. Eating more carbohydrate will increase your blood glucose level. Some health-care providers may recommend not taking additional bolus insulin unless you eat more than 15 grams of carbohydrate. Another blood glucose check would not be necessary when the additional food was eaten. If you did check 10 or 15 minutes after starting your meal, it would simply reveal that your blood glucose was rising. This is exactly what would be expected. Check with your health-care provider for your individual instructions.

Many pumps have a bolus calculator feature, which can be a big help in this situation. Your health-care provider sets the calculator based on your needs. The settings, entered by you or your health-care provider, include your blood glucose target range, an insulin-to-carbohydrate ratio for mealtime insulin, an insulin correction or sensitivity factor to bring your blood glucose back into target range, and your active insulin time (often set between 3 and 6 hours).

If you use the bolus calculator feature, it will take all these factors into account. It will tell you how much insulin is needed to cover a certain amount of carbohydrate and correct your blood glucose level if needed.

However, you should not take more correction insulin when you deliver the additional food bolus. This is called "stacking insulin," and it can put you at risk for a low blood glucose reaction. To understand the idea of stacking insulin, you have to consider your "insulin on board," the amount of insulin that is active in your body. Your premeal dose, or bolus, includes mealtime and often correction insulin if your blood glucose level is above your target before eating. As soon as you deliver a premeal dose, your pump tracks the insulin on board for you.

Most pumps use rapid-acting, or mealtime, insulin (aspart, lispro, or glulisine). Whether it's delivered by pump or injection, it works the same. Rapid-acting insulin's onset of action is about 10–15 minutes. Its effect peaks in about 1–2 hours, and its duration is about 3–4 hours.

Let's say you took a mealtime bolus of 10 units of insulin (8 units for carbohydrate and 2 units for correction). One hour after the bolus, about 8 units of insulin are still working in your body. So, if you took more correction insulin after the premeal bolus, you would be stacking: layering additional correction insulin on your previous dose. Most health-care providers recommend waiting 3 or more hours before delivering another correction bolus. Check with your health-care provider to determine what the best approach is for you.

Why Does a C-Peptide Test Matter?

| 've used an insulin pump for 4 1/2 years (and have been insulin dependent for 24 years). After I turned 65 years old, Medicare was paying for my insulin and pump supplies. Recently, though, Medicare denied payment, saying my C-peptide level doesn't meet its criteria. Why does Medicare use a C-peptide test to make this decision?

R. Y., Morton, IL

Jill Weisenberger, MS, RDN, CDE, responds: Medicare covers the cost of using a pump only for people with proven type 1 diabetes or those whose insulin production is extremely low. The goal of an insulin pump is to mimic the insulin secretion patterns of a person without diabetes. Insulin pumps help people with diabetes achieve tight blood glucose control, which helps prevent some of the complications of diabetes.

What to Know: Measuring C-peptide helps health-care providers determine how much insulin your pancreas produces. The insulin that comes from your pancreas starts off as a larger molecule called proinsulin. Proinsulin then splits into two pieces: insulin and C-peptide. Low C-peptide suggests there is little insulin production. Having no C-peptide indicates that you produce no insulin. (The insulin you inject or get with your pump is not associated with C-peptide.) It appears that Medicare denied coverage of the cost of your pump supplies because you produce more insulin than meets Medicare criteria for use of a pump.

Possible Solutions: As you know from the time before you had a pump, multiple daily injections (MDI) of insulin can also mimic a healthy pancreas. MDI requires that you take a long-acting insulin to provide some insulin 24 hours per day. Additionally, you will take rapid-acting insulin with meals and perhaps with snacks. Just as you adjust the amount of insulin your pump delivers, you can adjust the amount of rapid-acting insulin you inject to match your food intake. Many people, however, find a pump much more convenient and precise.

You might also ask your physician about taking another measure of your C-peptide level. It's possible that there was a laboratory error. Also, as your diabetes progresses, your C-peptide level may decrease.

Takeaways: Blood glucose control delays the onset and slows the progression of eye, nerve, and kidney damage. You should be able to achieve similar blood glucose levels using either MDI or an insulin pump. Medicare, of course, prefers the lower-cost insulin therapy, which is MDI.

Will Liposuction Affect My Insulin Absorption?

Can a person with diabetes who uses an insulin pump safely undergo liposuction surgery in the abdominal area? That's typically where the pump infusion set is inserted, so I wonder if the surgery would change the absorption of insulin.

S. B., Columbus, OH

Robert A. Gabbay, MD, PhD, responds: Once the area at which the liposuction was performed heals, you should be able to use it again for your insulin pump, but sometimes this can be tricky if there is a lot of scarring from the liposuction surgery. In that case, the scarring could continue to impair insulin absorption from the abdomen, and you would need to use a different site.

Liposuction can remove excess fat tissue. But people with diabetes should not confuse it in any way with bariatric surgery or traditional weight loss. Dropping pounds helps to improve insulin resistance, lower cholesterol, and lower blood pressure. Liposuction, however, does not change insulin resistance or result in these other health benefits.

Though the procedure is relatively safe, like all surgeries it does present risks for complications and even death. It is important that you have control of your blood glucose before undergoing any procedure. It's essential that you discuss your options with your diabetes-care team.

Can I Drive on Insulin?

I am a 74-year-old who has had diabetes for the past 20 years. I work part-time driving large trucks 3 1/2 days or more every week. I now take two pills a day. How am I going to be able to keep my Department of Transportation (DOT) license if I need to start using insulin? The exam states in large print not to use insulin. I sent a request to DOT in Washington for an exemption, but with the doctors they want me to see and the papers they want me to fill out, I'm not sure if it's worth it.

H. B., Woodburn, IN

Katie Hathaway, JD, Managing Director, Legal Advocacy, American Diabetes Association, responds: The situation you are facing is common and is why the American Diabetes Association has been fighting for so long on behalf of commercial drivers with diabetes.

For many years, federal law prohibited anyone with insulin-treated diabetes from operating a commercial motor vehicle in interstate commerce. Although some states permitted people using insulin to drive within their state, that only allowed a few people to maintain jobs in commercial driving.

These rules, dating back to the 1970s, were based on a misunderstanding of diabetes, especially how the disease is managed today. It is true that some people, because of the complications of diabetes, cannot safely drive a commercial vehicle. That is not true for most people. Fairness requires that each person be judged as an individual based on how diabetes affects him or her.

The American Diabetes Association worked for many years, through Congress and the administrative process, to eliminate this blanket ban. In 2003, we succeeded, and the Diabetes Exemption Program was born, establishing a system of individual assessment. This was a big step forward, but the program contained a provision that disqualified anyone who hadn't been driving a commercial vehicle while using insulin for the prior 3 years—and that meant almost no one could apply. This requirement was not necessary to ensure safety, as the program contained over 50 other safety provisions. So, the Association went back to Congress, and in the summer of 2005 a new law was signed eliminating the 3-year requirement.

The exemption program isn't perfect—it can take up to 6 months for an application to be processed, and sometimes longer than that for a final decision. The process involves an examination by an endocrinologist and either an ophthalmologist or an optometrist, and you will be asked to provide information about your diabetes, including any complications, hospitalizations, or history of hypoglycemia.

The good news is that since 2005, over 2,600 people with insulin-treated diabetes have been granted exemptions. Many of the people who received exemptions have type 2 diabetes and needed to begin using insulin. Prior to the Diabetes Exemption Program, these individuals had three choices: hope they lived in a state that offered medical waivers and could find a job that didn't require interstate driving; start a new career after years as a commercial driver; or jeopardize their health by ignoring their doctor's advice to begin using insulin.

We continue to fight to improve the system. Our goal is to eliminate the administrative burden of the Diabetes Exemption Program and replace it with a system for individual assessment that is done in the regular course of applying for DOT certification.

For more information about the American Diabetes Association's efforts in this area, please visit www.diabetes.org/CDL.

Is Insulin Less Effective in Transit?

I have a pump and use Humalog. I change the cartridge every 3 days and have noticed a drop-off in effectiveness on day three. When I traveled to Ireland for 12 days, I decided to change the cartridge every fourth day while I was there. I increased my boluses on day four, but could never catch up with my increased glucose readings. The insulin seemed to be at a 20–40% effectiveness.

Lilly or some other manufacturer must have on hand the degradation rate at different temperatures. I would assume the temperature of insulin in a pump in my pocket is somewhere between room temperature and body temperature. I realize that insulin is a complex animal, but any information would be helpful to making adjustments on day three or day four.

D. M.

Christy Parkin, MSN, RD, CDE, responds: Yes, insulin is a complex animal. It is a small protein that is particularly sensitive to environmental factors, especially temperature extremes. Although I do not know whether temperature was, in fact, the cause of your loss of insulin effectiveness, all of the insulin manufacturers warn against using insulin that has been exposed to temperatures higher than 86°F, either in the vial or in your insulin pump cartridge. The temperature of the insulin may exceed ambient temperature when the pump housing, cover, tubing, or sport case is exposed to sunlight or radiant heat. Another point to consider during your travels is that any unopened insulin you bring will need to be refrigerated at 36–46°F, and not exposed to any extreme heat, cold, or light. After the vial of insulin is open, it can be used for up to 28 days. However, there may be more going on than simply changes in insulin temperature.

Travel can make blood glucose control somewhat difficult because of the body's response to changes in time zones, sleeping patterns, eating schedule, activity level, and other factors. That's why extra blood glucose monitoring is recommended during travel. Also, it is not uncommon to notice a drop in effectiveness of insulin on day three of pump wear, which could be a site issue or an insulin issue. Changing sites every 2 days can be very helpful, although I realize that changing sites more often increases the cost of your supplies.

In your case, using your cartridge for an extra day (from 3 to 4 days), combined with international travel, may have contributed to your higher blood glucose levels. The main thing to remember is that it's important to check your blood glucose frequently while you are traveling so that you can make appropriate insulin adjustments. And, again, you need to protect your insulin from extreme temperatures. If you continue to have questions about the effectiveness of your insulin, I recommend that you contact the manufacturer. In the case of Humalog, contact the Lilly Answers Center at 1-800-LillyRx (1-800-545-5979).

Complications

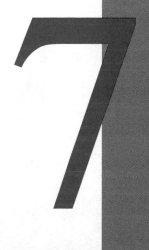

Will Little Issues Get Bigger?

I am a 61-year-old woman and I have been on insulin for 38 years. My A1C is usually a little over 7%.

Over the past year, it seems I always have some infection or problem: cataracts, bladder infection and interstitial cystitis, sinus infections, ingrown toenail, bursitis in an elbow and carpal tunnel in a hand, and root canals and two teeth pulled.

I'm worried that these small problems are the beginning of more serious things. What can I do to help with the obvious inflammation in my body?

Name Withheld

Janis McWilliams, RN, MSN, CDE, BC-ADM, responds:

What to Know: It is difficult not to worry when medical problems accumulate. As you are aware, diabetes puts you at greater risk for developing some conditions. Carpal tunnel syndrome is more common in women and people with diabetes. People with diabetes are more likely to develop cataracts at a younger age. Women, especially postmenopausal women, are more prone to develop urinary tract infections than men, and women with diabetes are at greater risk. Dental problems in diabetes are usually related to gum disease.

Sinus infections aren't necessarily related to diabetes, although if diabetes is not well controlled, the immune system can be weakened. People with diabetes do need to maintain good foot care, which includes cutting your toenails straight across. However, anyone can have ingrown toenails. There is no established link between diabetes and bursitis.

Possible Solutions: Some of your problems may be related to having diabetes. However, just getting older can also be a risk! None of us can stop aging, but there are some things that you can do to improve your chances of avoiding more problems. We know that well-controlled diabetes helps avoid complications. Enjoy as happy and active a lifestyle as you can, and try not to be discouraged by the medical bumps in the road.

Takeaways: You have had diabetes for a long time and seem to have reasonable control, judging by your A1C. However, the American Diabetes Association recommends keeping A1C below 7% for most people. Check with your health-care provider about how you can achieve your individual goal. A diabetes educator may also provide tips based on your lifestyle and treatment to help you tighten the target range for your blood glucose levels.

How Do I Help Someone Who Is Experiencing Hypoglycemia?

I work in a nursing home with several diabetic residents. Last week, one of our residents (a dialysis patient) had a blood glucose of 41 mg/dl. It was very unusual for him to have a low. He was somewhat responsive and drank 8 ounces of juice, then 8 ounces of chocolate Ensure. I had to keep my colleagues from adding sugar to the juice! Then, once the resident was stable, we fed him peanut butter crackers and he was fine. My peers and I are now reviewing what we could have done differently, and what we could use in the future if we didn't have juice. Is cake frosting recommended? Is there anything else we should know?

E. P., Henrico County, VA

Janis McWilliams, RN, MSN, CDE, BC-ADM, responds: It is a great idea to review treatment of patients to develop best practices for the future. Hypoglycemia (low blood glucose) is defined as a blood glucose of less than 70 mg/dl. The recommended treatment for hypoglycemia is to consume 15–20 grams of carbohydrate, then recheck blood glucose in 15 minutes. If the level is still below 70 mg/dl, treat again with 15 grams of carbohydrate, and so on until glucose is 70 mg/dl or above.

Here are a few examples of carbohydrate-containing foods and drinks to give to a conscious person experiencing a low: three to five glucose tablets, 1/2 cup (4 ounces) of fruit juice, 1 cup of nonfat milk, or 1/2 cup (4 ounces) of non-diet soda. Whatever initial carbohydrate source is used, it should not include fat or protein, both of which may slow down the rate of absorption. Both Ensure and many cake frostings contain fat and, therefore, are not the best choices. However, once a person's glucose is higher than 70 mg/dl, and it's not time for a meal, half a turkey sandwich is a good choice. (Peanut butter isn't recommended for someone with kidney disease because it's high in phosphorus and potassium.)

You are right not to add sugar to the juice, as that could well result in hyperglycemia (high blood glucose). Also, note that orange juice is high in potassium and is usually restricted for someone on a renal diet, in which case I would recommend apple juice.

If hypoglycemia causes someone to be unconscious, the best treatment—if you don't have IV access—is glucagon, a hormone that raises blood glucose and that is administered intramuscularly or under the skin as a shot. Once the glucagon injection is given, be sure to turn the patient onto his or her side, as glucagon may cause some patients to vomit. It would be a good idea to add glucagon to your facility's emergency cart. Never give an unconscious person food or drink; it may cause choking and difficulty breathing.

Although your patient has infrequent hypoglycemia, you should be aware that as kidney function declines, insulin can last longer and be unpredictable in its action. Some patients on dialysis have frequent hypoglycemia, which is difficult to predict.

Diabetes Forecast publishes an annual consumer guide to diabetes supplies, including products for treating lows. The most recent guide is available at www.diabetesforecast.org/consumerguide.

How Can I Spot DKA?

I recently found myself in the hospital with a diagnosis of diabetic ketoacidosis. It was a complete shock. Just an awareness of what DKA is, how serious it can be, and what its symptoms are could help keep someone from getting a costly hospital bill and, more importantly, a potentially deadly diagnosis.

M. H., Manhattan, KS

Paris Roach, MD, responds: It's essential for everyone with type 1 diabetes to know the risk factors for and the symptoms of diabetic ketoacidosis (DKA) and how to prevent it. (DKA can develop in people with type 2 diabetes, but it's less common.) The two main causes of DKA are interruption of insulin treatment (missing insulin injections or failure of an insulin pump system) and severe illness, such as the flu with fever or even a heart attack or stroke.

Insulin controls the production of ketones, the substances that build up in the bloodstream and cause DKA, so if someone with type 1 diabetes stops taking insulin, DKA can result. During an illness, the body produces stress hormones, which counteract insulin action to such an extent that DKA can develop. High blood glucose levels result, leading to excessive urination and dehydration, which in turn push blood glucose and ketones to even higher levels. Some people incorrectly assume that if they're sick and not eating, they shouldn't take insulin, but this will result in rapid development of DKA. That's why it's important to work with your care provider early during an illness to determine the best way to avoid interruption of insulin treatment. Dehydration that occurs because of vomiting, inability to eat and drink, and high glucose and ketone levels can also contribute to rapid worsening of DKA.

The symptoms of DKA include nausea, vomiting, abdominal pain, dry mouth, thirst, and excessive urination. In advanced stages of DKA, a rapid, deep breathing pattern develops, and the breath takes on a fruity odor. A decreased level of consciousness is particularly ominous and should prompt a call for emergency medical services.

The best way to prevent DKA is to check your urine ketones when your blood glucose is persistently high (greater than 250 mg/dl) and not responding normally to additional insulin, especially if you're sick. Urine ketone test strips are available at pharmacies; blood ketone meters and strips are available, but are less common. If you have persistently elevated urine ketone levels, call your health-care provider. Consider whether your insulin may have gone bad because of exposure to heat or cold. Check your blood glucose and ketones frequently when you're sick, and keep taking your long-acting insulin along with small doses of short-acting insulin to correct high blood glucose as directed by your health-care provider. DKA can develop rapidly, so it's very important to check ketones early, to seek professional medical advice, and to go for emergency care promptly if your blood glucose and ketone levels are not responding to treatment. If you're persistently nauseated or vomiting and can't drink fluids to stay hydrated, you should call your care provider immediately. Although these symptoms can be due to an underlying illness, they can also signal the development of DKA.

All people with type 1 diabetes should have on hand a reliable means for measuring urine ketones. When in doubt, check your ketones—it's easy and inexpensive, and it provides the critical information needed to prevent DKA.

Will Pregnancy Put Me at Risk?

| am the 33-year-old mom of a healthy 2-year-old boy, and I have type 1 diabetes. I've been told by two doctors that pregnancy decreases the life expectancy of a woman with diabetes. The thought really upsets me. Is this true?

Name Withheld

Paris Roach, MD, responds:

What to Know: Women with type 1 or type 2 diabetes can have uneventful pregnancies, healthy babies, and normal healthy lives after their babies are born. Pregnant women with diabetes, however, may have additional health risks compared with those without diabetes.

Preexisting retinopathy (diabetic eye problems) can worsen during pregnancy, as can preexisting nephropathy (diabetic kidney disease). The development of advanced kidney disease during pregnancy could potentially decrease the life span of the mother, especially if she has to undergo dialysis for a long period of time. The presence of vascular disease (coronary artery disease and/or cerebrovascular disease, the cause of strokes and ministrokes, or TIAs), which is more common in women with diabetes, confers especially high risk for a pregnant woman because pregnancy places a high demand on the cardiovascular system. Additionally, poor glucose control during pregnancy can lead to maternal complications during pregnancy and/or delivery that could affect the long-term health of the mother.

Find Out More: The best way to limit risks to mother and baby in diabetic pregnancies is to plan, plan, plan. Consult your care team if you are even considering trying to become pregnant in the next year or so. If your blood glucose isn't under excellent control, start now. Undergo appropriate evaluations for diabetic complications and cardiovascular disease. Have your thyroid hormone levels checked, as adequate thyroid hormone is important for both maternal health and fetal development. Your care provider should also monitor you for the development of thyroid problems after delivery, which are especially common in women with type 1 diabetes. If your blood pressure is elevated, get on a baby-safe treatment regimen and have a frank discussion with your health-care provider about the pregnancy risks conferred by high blood pressure.

Eat healthfully, engage in moderate exercise, and take the appropriate vitamins. Take time to take care of yourself before you become pregnant so that diabetic complications and other risks can be discussed and dealt with before, instead of during, pregnancy.

Takeaway: If you came through your pregnancy without worsening of diabetes complications or cardiovascular events, there would seem to be no evidence that pregnancy has affected your long-term health.

What Are the Basic Steps of Foot Care?

I am 20 years old, and I have been diabetic for almost 10 years now with no foot problems. However, I always read about people with diabetes having to take care of their feet, and it scares me to think that one day I may have to get a foot amputated. I play tennis very often and have many calluses on my feet—do I need to be worried?

C. P.

Lee J. Sanders, DPM, responds: Your question is an important one. Simply put, healthy foot care habits that are developed early in life make a big difference in later years. Foot inspection should be an important part of your daily routine and diabetes self-management. Early recognition of uncomplicated conditions can prevent the development of more serious complications. You should look for the following signs and symptoms, comparing one foot with the other:

1. A change in the size or shape of the foot
2. A change in skin color (becoming red or blue)
3. A change in skin temperature (warmer or cooler)
4. An open area of skin (blister or sore) with or without drainage
5. An ingrown toenail
6. Structural deformities of the foot (hammertoes or bunions)
7. Corns or calluses
8. Pain, burning, tingling, or numbness in your feet

Acute changes should be promptly reported to your podiatrist or the health-care provider taking care of your diabetes. Regular professional foot care is advised for treatment of your calluses. Treating these conditions yourself is ill-advised. Daily use of an emollient (cream or lotion) is helpful for dry skin care (and reminds you to look at your feet).

Selection of footwear should be appropriate for the occasion. Your feet should be measured and shoes should be properly fitted by an experienced shoe fitter. Athletic shoes are generally designed for specific sports activities. Make sure that your tennis shoes fit well, are comfortable, and are in good condition. Make sure to wear athletic socks. Socks made with a blend of acrylic and natural fibers are best for wicking moisture away from the skin.

An annual foot exam is recommended for identification of conditions that may require further investigation or treatment. Prevention of foot complications is the key objective. Amputation is not an inevitable consequence of diabetes.

Can Diabetes Cause Burning in the Feet?

M y friend was recently diagnosed with diabetes. He complains that his feet feel very hot from time to time. Is this related to diabetes?

N. C., Port Elizabeth, South Africa

Lee J. Sanders, DPM, responds: A hot or burning sensation in the feet, especially in middle-aged and older people, could be caused by small fiber neuropathy (damage to nerves). Diabetes is the most common cause of this condition; symptoms typically start with burning, tingling, and numbness in the toes and feet. Even though your friend was only recently diagnosed with diabetes, if it is the cause of the burning in his feet, then he has probably had impaired glucose tolerance for years now. Peripheral neuropathy—in the feet, legs, and hands—and peripheral vascular disease, which can be caused by diabetes, are potential culprits, and your friend should see his podiatrist or medical doctor for a comprehensive diabetic foot screening examination.

Though this sensation is not uncommon in people with diabetes, hot or burning feet can have many other causes. Since your friend says his feet feel very hot from time to time, but not all the time, he and his doctor should rule out other causes. A person's occupation, activity, and footwear are frequently responsible for hot feet. A postal worker, police officer, or construction worker might experience hot or burning feet because of prolonged periods of standing as well as exposure to hot temperatures on the ground. Running or playing basketball, golf, or tennis on a hot day could also cause this sensation. Shoes, especially those that are enclosed and/or made with synthetic materials, can cause hot, sweaty feet, which in turn can cause a burning sensation. Socks may also contribute to this condition.

Another common cause of burning feet is athlete's foot (*tinea pedis*). Some less common causes include alcoholism, chronic kidney failure, peripheral arterial disease, tarsal tunnel syndrome, Morton's neuroma, vitamin deficiency, HIV or AIDS, complex regional pain syndrome, and gastric bypass surgery.

Your friend should discuss this concern with his podiatrist, family doctor, or endocrinologist. A change in footwear or treatment of athlete's foot may be all that is needed to remedy this ailment. In the meantime, the following recommendations may be helpful:

- Alternate shoes every other day to air them out.
- If weather permits, wear an enclosed protective sandal to allow your feet to breathe.
- Change your socks often, especially after exercise. Socks made from COOLMAX fiber or a blend of polyester fibers are recommended

because they more effectively wick sweat away from the feet and cool them down.

- Wear shower shoes when using public showers or pools.
- Use a medicated foot powder to absorb excess moisture and to treat athlete's foot fungus.

What Causes Charcot Foot?

What is the cause of Charcot foot in people with diabetes, and how can it be prevented?

A. B., South Pasadena, CA

Lee J. Sanders, DPM, responds: The Charcot foot is a rare, potentially serious condition that occurs in some people with diabetes. There is no single cause for the development of this condition. However, two important factors are minor trauma and the loss of sensation in your feet—nerve damage that is referred to as peripheral sensory neuropathy. Neuropathy is a common complication of diabetes, seen in people with both type 1 and type 2 diabetes. The earliest sign of the Charcot foot may be a sudden and unexpected change in the appearance of your foot or ankle, characterized by redness, swelling, and warmth. You may have no recollection of injury.

X-rays of the foot may initially look perfectly normal, or there may be only subtle changes that can be easily missed. This is the most important stage of the Charcot foot for the physician to recognize the problem and to start treatment immediately. Treatment is aimed at offloading the foot, to prevent further foot fractures and dislocations, with immobilization in a cast or brace. It is extremely important to stay off of the affected foot until inflammation subsides and the foot is stable. Sometimes there is collapse of the arch with the development of bony deformity, a "rocker-bottom foot," with formation of an open sore (ulcer) on the bottom of the foot. Your doctor will first need to confirm the diagnosis by eliminating other conditions that might have a similar appearance, such as infection or gout. Diabetic foot specialists will apply a non-weight-bearing total contact cast and monitor the condition closely. Serial x-rays are taken to evaluate the healing of fractures and dislocations of one or more joints. Immobilization in a cast can take 3 months or longer. Patients are often transitioned from a non-weight-bearing cast to a removable walking brace, and then to a special shoe. In most cases, patients can be treated with nonsurgical care; in the most difficult cases, surgery may be necessary.

Treatment of the Charcot foot is often prolonged, challenging, and frustrating. If you are at high risk—if you have peripheral neuropathy with loss of protective sensation in your feet—you should know the implications of sensory loss, as well as the importance of diabetes self-management. Foot inspection should be an important part of your daily routine. Compare one foot with the other and look for changes in size or shape. Is one foot swollen? Are there changes in the color or temperature of the skin? If you notice any of these changes, call your podiatrist, diabetes specialist, or family physician, and request to be seen as soon as possible.

What Can I Do for Numb, Painful Feet and Legs?

My husband was diagnosed with diabetes almost a year ago. At first he was experiencing numbness in his feet. Over the past few months, he began having pain as well, sometimes as far up his leg as his calf. What can we do to help these symptoms? I have read that vitamin E and even flaxseed oil are good for the circulation. Would those be helpful?

Name Withheld

Lee J. Sanders, DPM, responds: Your husband may have a condition that should be treated with doctor-prescribed medication, and a proper diagnosis is vital to determining how to treat what he is experiencing. The likely cause of his symptoms is either peripheral arterial disease (PAD), which is due to poor circulation, or diabetic peripheral neuropathy (DPN), due to nerve damage. Here are some questions that would help your health-care provider with a diagnosis: Does your husband have pain in his legs when he walks? (If so, how far can he walk before he must stop to rest?) Do his feet appear red or blue in color when they are lowered, and does the redness disappear with elevation of his legs? Are his feet and legs cold? Does he hang his leg over the side of the bed at night to relieve pain? Is only one leg affected by pain, and is this leg swollen, warm to the touch, and reddish-brown in color? A "Yes" to any of these questions may indicate peripheral vascular disease, and your husband should see his doctor immediately if that is the case.

If he is not having any of the above signs and symptoms, then he may be suffering from neuropathy. DPN is an important quality-of-life issue for half of all people with diabetes. The pain is often described by patients as tingling, burning, sharp, shooting, and lightning-like. Other unpleasant symptoms include numbness, feelings of feet and legs being "asleep," or prickling or crawling sensations. However, not all peripheral neuropathy is caused by diabetes. The diagnosis of DPN can be made only after a careful clinical examination. All people with diabetes should be screened annually for DPN.

Although there is currently no cure for this complication of diabetes, optimal glucose control helps to prevent DPN. Several studies suggest that avoiding extreme fluctuations in blood glucose helps as well. It's also recommended that people with either condition improve cholesterol levels and blood pressure, do not smoke, and avoid excessive alcohol consumption. Many people will require a medication to manage their painful symptoms; avoid trying an unproven method or remedy, such as vitamin E or flaxseed oil. (People with diabetes should always check with their health-care provider before taking any supplement to make sure it doesn't interfere with their medications.) A proper diagnosis needs to be established before your husband can move forward with the right treatment.

How Do I Fight
Toenail Fungus?

What can you tell me about the dreaded toe fungus? It seems to develop very slowly and can get vicious! I've heard it can get all through the system if not treated. Just what can happen? More important, is there a way to avoid it, besides the regular foot care, dry feet, no bare feet, etc.? Is there an over-the-counter cream that can cure the fungus before it gets so bad that oral meds are needed?

A. P., Ashdown, AR

Lee J. Sanders, DPM, responds: The medical term for the toenail fungus that you refer to is onychomycosis. This condition is a ubiquitous infection of the toenails caused by a mold or yeast. Onychomycosis is often associated with a chronic athlete's foot condition. A 2006 study published in the journal *Acta Dermato-Venereologica* reported that 22% of patients with diabetes have toenail onychomycosis. Many people live with this condition for their entire lives; however, onychomycosis can negatively impact your quality of life. In addition to the cosmetic effects, the toenail fungus can cause nail deformity, pain or discomfort while wearing shoes, odor, or recurrent ingrown toenails. In people with diabetes, onychomycosis can lead to serious foot complications such as foot ulcers and infections. Although topical antifungal medications are effective for treatment of fungus infection of the skin (*tinea pedis*), they are relatively ineffective for infection of the toenails. The medication is unable to penetrate the nail plate to get to the fungus. For some people, oral antifungal medications can provide a cure for onychomycosis, when used appropriately.

A clinical cure frequently takes close to a year, and recurrence of the infection is common. You should discuss treatment options with your physician or podiatrist. Prior to treatment with an oral antifungal medication, your healthcare provider should perform a careful medical history and a visual inspection of your nails, perform a fungal culture, and order a blood test to determine whether your liver function is normal. The use of laser treatment for fungus nails is controversial.

Good foot care is essential for all people with diabetes. You should keep your feet clean and dry, wear shower shoes when bathing or when at the local swimming pool or health club, and wear socks made of a blend of absorbent fibers. Acrylic fiber socks transport moisture more efficiently from the surface of the foot than do cotton socks. Remember that inadequate laundering of clothing (socks) can be a source of reinfection following therapy for onychomycosis and athlete's foot.

Does Diabetes Cause Glaucoma?

Can it be shown that diabetes frequently causes glaucoma? If so, what is the connection?

G. K., Lutz, FL

Janis McWilliams, RN, MSN, CDE, BC-ADM, responds: Glaucoma has long been considered one of the eye complications that can affect people with diabetes. One rare form, neovascular glaucoma, is definitely associated with diabetes. Another type, open-angle glaucoma, is much more common. Scientists are "quite divided," however, over whether open-angle glaucoma has a particular link to diabetes, says Alon Harris, PhD, director of clinical research at the Indiana University School of Medicine's Glick Eye Institute.

What to Know: Glaucoma occurs when there is a gradual increase in the normal fluid pressure inside the eyes. The increased pressure can damage the optic nerve, causing vision loss. Glaucoma is an insidious disease, because there are no symptoms until there is a loss of peripheral (side) vision. If glaucoma is left untreated, the result can be complete vision loss. The longer someone has had diabetes, the chances of developing glaucoma increase. The risk for glaucoma in everyone grows with age.

Find Out More: About 90% of all people with glaucoma have open-angle glaucoma. This condition is characterized by a slow clogging of the drainage canals that typically prevent too much liquid from building up in the eye. Too much liquid results in increased eye pressure that can damage the optic nerve. The less common neovascular glaucoma that tends to be associated with diabetes occurs when new, abnormal blood vessels grow on the iris, the colored part of the eye. These blood vessels block the normal flow of fluid out of the eye, raising the eye pressure.

Possible Solutions: Treatment of glaucoma can include special eye drops, laser procedures, medications, or surgery. Surgery and laser treatments are directed at improving the eye's drainage of fluid.

Takeaways: Early detection is the key to treating glaucoma successfully and keeping the disease from worsening. It is important to have a glaucoma test as part of your yearly dilated eye exam, especially if you have diabetes. Also, maintaining glucose control should lower the risk of complications, including those of the eye.

How Do I Handle Diverticulitis?

How do I handle diverticulitis? I have found next to no information about how someone with type 2 diabetes on insulin should deal with bouts of diverticulitis. Please help!

M. M., Tumwater, WA

Janis McWilliams, RN, MSN, CDE, BC-ADM, responds: Diverticula are small, bulging pouches found mostly in your large intestine. These are thought to result in part from a diet high in processed foods and too low in fiber. However, diverticulosis (the development of these pouches) is a very common condition, and the incidence increases as we age. When one or more of these pouches becomes inflamed or infected, diverticulitis develops.

Diverticulitis symptoms include abdominal pain, tenderness, fever, nausea, and constipation or diarrhea. The pain can feel like appendicitis, except it is usually in the lower left side of your abdomen instead of the lower right side.

Treatment depends on the severity of symptoms, but usually starts with a liquid or low-fiber diet and antibiotics. This can lead to difficulties for people on insulin, as you mentioned. Instead of eating a diet high in fiber and whole grains, whole fruits, and vegetables—the usual ingredients for a healthy diet— these foods need to be avoided to rest the colon until the infection heals. This change in eating will usually lead to a change in insulin requirements to best manage blood glucose.

It is impossible for me to make specific recommendations, as each patient is different. However, if you take a premixed insulin such as 70/30 or 75/25, it would likely be better to take a basal insulin and be able to give premeal rapid-acting shots based on what you are going to eat and the total carbohydrate content. If you are on a liquid diet, you need to be sure that it includes carbohydrate for energy. Instead of sugar-free soda, gelatin, and popsicles, switch to choices with calories and carbohydrate. Certain fruit juices without pulp are also allowed. Your diabetes educator can help you match your carbohydrate amount with your insulin dose.

It is good to remember that although a low-fiber diet is the treatment for diverticulitis, once the symptoms are gone, you should try to gradually increase the fiber in your diet to best avoid another attack. Getting regular exercise and drinking plenty of fluids also help to avoid a recurrence.

What Is "Diabetic Stomach"?

My niece takes an oral medicine for diabetes. At least once a week, she throws up at night. The doctor calls it "diabetic stomach." I have never heard of this, and I have had diabetes for 36 years.

What could be the cause of her stomach problems, and what foods may be causing flare-ups?

G. S., Philadelphia, PA

Roger P. Austin, MS, RPh, CDE, responds: The medical term for the condition your niece's doctor calls "diabetic stomach" is gastroparesis. Diabetes can cause alterations of peristalsis, the normal contractions of the stomach and intestines that move food along the digestive tract. In patients with diabetes and gastroparesis, this movement is slowed, causing food to be retained in the stomach for longer than normal. This sometimes can cause nausea and vomiting.

High blood glucose levels (hyperglycemia) contribute to this slowing of both stomach and intestinal movement. If the hyperglycemia occurs over a prolonged period of time, it can cause damage to nerves that supply the stomach, a condition called autonomic neuropathy, which worsens the gastroparesis and makes it very difficult to control. High blood glucose is the source of the underlying problem of gastroparesis. However, certain foods, such as fatty foods, caffeine, and chocolate, can relax the lower esophageal sphincter (the valve between the esophagus and the stomach), making the gastroparesis symptoms worse. The most effective treatment for your niece, if the onset of her gastroparesis is recent, is for her to aggressively lower her blood glucose levels to her target ranges and to keep her A1C under 7%. Working with a dietitian can help your niece find an eating plan—often involving smaller, more regular meals, thorough chewing, and limits on high-fat and high-fiber foods—that may help. Medications and gastric pacing devices are also possible treatments. For some people with diabetes and gastroparesis who are only on oral medications, achieving these targets may require the use of insulin.

How to Treat
Diabetic Diarrhea?

| have a problem that I never see addressed. I've had type 1 diabe-
tes for 36 years and been diagnosed as having diabetic diarrhea.
Numerous tests have ruled out all other gastrointestinal problems.
Is there any treatment for this problem?

Name Withheld

Janis McWilliams, RN, MSN, CDE, BC-ADM, responds: People with diabetes may, of course, develop diarrhea for a variety of reasons, just like anyone else. Diarrhea is a symptom of many diseases such as viral or bacterial infections, celiac disease, irritable bowel syndrome, and Crohn's disease. It is a side effect of some medications, such as metformin, and some sugar-free sweeteners can cause diarrhea in some people.

However, diarrhea can also be a symptom of a type of autonomic neuropathy or nerve damage. This is what is known as diabetic diarrhea. Although this condition is not uncommon, the diagnosis is usually made only after a detailed history and diagnostic tests reveal no other cause for the diarrhea.

Unlike the more widely known peripheral sensory neuropathy, which affects the hands and feet, autonomic neuropathy damages the nerves that control involuntary activities of the body. More commonly known types of autonomic neuropathy include erectile dysfunction and orthostatic (or postural) hypotension, the feeling of light-headedness or dizziness you get from standing after lying or sitting down.

Diabetic diarrhea occurs usually at night, is watery and painless, and can be associated with fecal incontinence. Bouts of diarrhea can be episodic, along with intermittently normal bowel habits or even alternating with periods of constipation.

The treatment for diabetic diarrhea is individualized, but it generally starts with antidiarrheal agents such as Lomotil (a combination of diphenoxylate and atropine) or Imodium (loperamide). High-fiber foods or bulk-forming laxatives such as Metamucil may help decrease the symptoms. As with all neuropathies, good glucose control is important in controlling the symptoms.

Your health-care provider may order antispasmodic medicines to decrease the frequency of bowel movements. If bacterial overgrowth in the intestines is thought to be present, antibiotics may be ordered. Medications like clonidine or octreotide, which have other primary uses but have been shown to help diarrhea, can be used in more advanced cases that do not respond to other treatments. Although your primary care doctor or endocrinologist can initiate treatment for diabetic diarrhea, a referral to a gastroenterologist may be indicated when standard therapies are ineffective.

Does Diabetes Cause Trigger Finger?

I recently had surgery to release a condition called trigger finger in my middle finger and thumb. My doctor said this is a common malady in people with diabetes. Why?

M. D., Buffalo, NY

Christy Parkin, MSN, RN, CDE, responds: Trigger finger is a musculoskeletal condition that affects the tendons and ligaments in the fingers or thumb. In trigger finger, a finger or thumb gets stuck in a bent position and then straightens with a snap—like a trigger being pulled and released. In severe cases, the finger may become locked in a bent position.

What to Know: The cause of trigger finger is usually unknown. The condition is more common in women than men and occurs most often in people between the ages of 40 and 60 years, sometimes after activities that strain the hand. People with certain medical problems, including diabetes, hypothyroidism, and rheumatoid arthritis, are more likely to develop trigger finger. The condition affects 2–3% of the population but 10–20% of those with diabetes. Its presence is associated with age and duration of diabetes, not with blood glucose control. In people with type 1 diabetes, trigger finger has been linked to carpal tunnel syndrome.

Find Out More: Signs and symptoms of trigger finger usually start without any injury and may progress from mild to severe. They include:

- Finger stiffness, particularly in the morning
- Pain when bending or straightening your finger
- A popping or clicking sensation as you move your finger
- Tenderness or a bump at the base of the affected finger
- The finger catching or locking in a bent position, then popping straight
- The finger locking in a bent position, which you can't straighten

Possible Solutions: Treatment varies depending on trigger finger's severity and duration. Rest, splinting, physical therapy, and avoiding repetitive gripping may alleviate mild or infrequent symptoms. For more serious cases, nonsteroidal anti-inflammatory drugs (NSAIDs), steroid injections, or surgery may be necessary.

Takeaways: Trigger finger is not a dangerous condition, although it certainly can affect your quality of life. The goal of surgery is to release the tendon when symptoms become severe and don't respond to other treatments. This minor operation can provide permanent relief.

Can Diabetes Cause Persistent Bladder Infections?

For the past year, I have had multiple bladder infections (three in the past 30 days), most often with very minimal symptoms. I have been told by my urologist that my infections have nothing to do with poor hygiene, but with organisms that my immune system does not seem to fight very well.

I take antibiotics to treat the infections, and cranberry juice supplements and probiotics to help prevent the infections, and I have not had a sexual partner for some time.

I know that people with diabetes, and women in general, are more susceptible to urinary tract infections, but wonder how common it is for women with diabetes to have so many infections. I am also concerned about possible kidney damage due to asymptomatic infections that may be untreated for weeks or months at a time. I would appreciate any information you could give me on the subject.

Name Withheld

Frank Rodriguez, MD, responds: First and foremost, you need to make sure you have blood glucose control, or you will continue to have these problems.

Second, symptomatic cystitis and bladder problems in people with diabetes will occur, and it may be useful to schedule periodic urinalysis and/or bacterial cultures to keep the problem from recurring.

Third, cranberry derivatives are only useful intermittently. If used to prevent cystitis, they should only be used 1 day out of the week. The cranberry products inhibit the common intestinal bacteria *E. coli*'s ability to attach to membran es in your bladder—that is a short-term effect. Beyond 48 hours, the *E. coli* adapt to the active agent, and then you just have expensive urine.

Fourth, are you pre- or postmenopausal? If you have already gone through menopause, then you need local estrogens to keep the epithelium, the layer of tissues around the bladder (and other organs, including skin), healthy and resistant to pathogens.

Try logging a urinary diary. Chances are good that you may not be urinating frequently enough. Also, you mention that you're not sexually active, but this can be an issue for some people. Partners of sexually active women should use condoms. Everyone thinks of the diagnosis of diabetes in a woman with recurrent bladder and vaginal yeast infections, but they forget that the partner may have chronic prostatitis, meaning that a man with diabetes may be depositing glucose-laden semen in the vaginal channel.

Finally, always ask your health-care provider about getting an HIV test if you have recurrent cases of urinary tract infection. Rule out HIV and then move on.

If these tips don't address your problem, a urogynecologist should be able to help you get to the root of the issue.

Do Recurrent Boils Have Anything to Do with Diabetes?

am a 43-year-old woman and I was diagnosed with type 1 diabetes 2 years ago. I've always had pretty good skin, but in the past year I've had a problem with boils in my groin area. My job is very stressful at times, and I think this has something to do with when they surface. I've noticed they usually rear their ugly heads between ovulation and my period, and at a time when I'm stressed out and eating poorly too. My gynecologist has prescribed me antibiotics to treat them twice already this year. Can you please tell me what the connection is between boils and diabetes, and how best to care for them?

Name Withheld

Belinda Childs, APRN, MN, BC-ADM, CDE, responds: Skin abscesses, also known as boils, are more common in people with uncontrolled diabetes. They are usually caused by bacteria, typically *Staphylococcus aureus* or *Streptococcus*, but the abscesses can also be caused by other bacteria. For example, MRSA (methicillin-resistant *Staphylococcus aureus*) is a dangerous bacteria that can initially look like a boil. It is important that the boils be evaluated by a health-care provider and the right antibiotic prescribed. You can develop blood infections from untreated abscesses. *Staphylococcus aureus* is the most common cause of infections at insulin pump needle sites.

Bacteria flourish in moist, dark, warm areas of the body, including the groin and underarm areas. You can get an abscess or boil in any location. We know that high blood glucose levels, even for short periods of time, can delay healing and increase the risk of infection. Stress, whether emotional or physical (including menstruation), can also lower your immunity and increase the likelihood that an infection will develop. Yeast and fungal infections are more common in people with uncontrolled diabetes too.

Keeping your blood glucose level as close to normal as possible will help reduce the frequency of the abscesses. Talk to your pharmacist about a strong antibacterial soap. Finally, even though it may be embarrassing, always talk to your health-care provider about any unusual skin infections.

Could This Be an Allergy?

I was recently diagnosed with type 1 diabetes, and shortly after I was released from the hospital, I started to develop a severely itchy rash.

Mostly it's located on my back, legs, chest, and stomach. The bumps are like hives and it itches horribly, enough to keep me from sleeping at night despite repeated applications of topical Benadryl, hydrocortisone, lotions, etc. I have tried everything, including a steroid cream that my doctor prescribed. She also prescribed a round of oral steroids, to no avail. I have heard that it is possible to have an allergic reaction to the insulin. It's the only medication that I take on a regular basis. Is this my problem?

K. E., Wichita, KS

Belinda Childs, APRN, MN, CDE, BC-ADM, responds: It is possible to have an insulin allergy, but it is rare today, now that we have human recombinant insulin and its analogs. Insulin allergy occurs in less than 1% of people. The typical reaction is a wheal and flare (like a hive) at the injection site. It is very rare to develop a rash and itch, or any more severe type of reaction. Usually, if someone has an allergy to insulin, the insulin also does not perform its job as well.

In most cases, the allergy is actually a reaction to the preservative in the insulin, not the insulin itself. A change in brand or type may help verify that it is not the insulin that is causing your reaction.

More common causes of rashes are new lotions, skin or laundry soap, clothing items, or other new irritants. Did you receive antibiotics or other medications besides insulin in the hospital? When did you first notice the rash? I would encourage you to think of the other things that may have been new or different around the time that you developed diabetes.

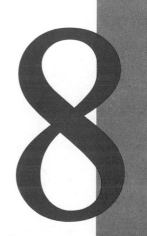

Miscellaneous Questions

How Do I Raise My HDL?

My HDL "good" cholesterol is 50 mg/dl and I was told to bring it up. How do I do this? I was told to drink 4 ounces of red wine at night. How else can I increase my HDL?

S. C.

Robert A. Gabbay, MD, PhD, responds: You bring up a very important question for people with diabetes—the role of cholesterol in reducing the risk for cardiovascular disease. HDL (the "good" cholesterol) can help lower your risk of heart disease, but it is often difficult to increase HDL levels on your own. One way to do it is through exercise. Red wine also seems to have some beneficial effect on HDL levels, but physicians generally do not ask people to start drinking wine if they are not already doing so (extra calories being one of the downsides). Medications can sometimes be helpful as well—the "fibrates" (fenofibrate and gemfibrozil) and niacin all can increase HDL cholesterol, particularly when triglyceride levels are high. Most important, controlling your blood glucose and lowering your A1C (an estimate of average blood glucose over the previous 2–3 months) can also raise your HDL and lower your triglycerides—one more reason to strive for blood glucose control.

Finally, we should not forget how important LDL (the "bad" cholesterol) is in determining cardiovascular risk. Statins like atorvastatin, simvastatin, or pravastatin are very effective in lowering LDL cholesterol. The goal for LDL cholesterol is usually less than 100 mg/dl, but if you already have heart disease, LDL of less than 70 mg/dl is probably best. We are finding out that these drugs (statins) lower the risk of heart attacks and strokes not only by lowering LDL but also because they seem to stabilize plaques in the arteries, making them less likely to rupture and cause heart attacks. Statins are among the most effective medications at lowering the risk of heart disease. Of course, avoiding too many saturated fats, not smoking, and adopting a healthy meal plan as recommended by the American Diabetes Association are important steps as well. Finally, exercise, as mentioned above, is another key piece of cardiovascular health. Some people with diabetes will also benefit from taking a daily aspirin, but you should consult with your health-care provider first.

Are Omega-3s Safe?

often see recommendations for eating more "heavy" fish (e.g., swordfish, tuna, mackerel) as a heart-healthy practice. I have a 2-year-old son and had been warned not to feed a child too much of these fish because of the mercury content.

There are other ways to enrich a child's diet with DHA or omega-3s such as enriched milk products, yogurt, and even infant formula. I would do just about anything to prevent type 1 diabetes in my child; however, I am not willing to risk mercury toxicity.

S. S.

Henry Rodriguez, MD, responds: There is no conclusive proof of the relationship between omega-3 fatty acid intake and a reduced risk of type 1 diabetes—rather, the data that have been collected show an association between the two, but not proof of cause and effect. We also have supportive data in animal models of type 1 diabetes. Relevant studies, including the TrialNet NIP (Nutritional Intervention to Prevent Type 1 Diabetes) study, have investigated the question prospectively.

There are potential risks of excess mercury, particularly with younger children. The U.S. Food and Drug Administration (FDA) recommends that young children avoid shark, swordfish, king mackerel, and tilefish, which are high in mercury. For further information about the risks of mercury in fish and shellfish, you can call the FDA's food information line toll-free at 1-888-SAFEFOOD or visit the FDA's "Food" web page at www.fda.gov/Food/. For information about the safety of locally caught fish and shellfish, visit the Environmental Protection Agency's "Fish Advisories" web page or contact your state or local health department. You are correct that there are safer alternative sources that can provide omega-3s. Other kinds of fatty fish that are high in omega-3 fatty acids include lake trout, salmon, and herring. Omega-3 supplements, like DHA, and soybean products are also options.

Given our current level of knowledge, I recommend following nutritional guidelines from the American Academy of Pediatrics, which is in accordance with the American Heart Association (AHA) in recommending an adequate intake of omega-3 fatty acids, and with both the AHA and the U.S. Food and Drug Administration in designating seafood as an important component of a healthy diet. The AHA guidelines recommend eating fish, particularly fatty fish, at least two times (two servings) a week. One serving is 3.5 ounces cooked, or about 3/4 cup of flaked fish.

Why Does Hot Yoga Raise My Number?

I am a 62-year-old woman with type 2 diabetes; my A1Cs range from 6.0 to 6.7%. I started Bikram (hot) yoga recently, and I really enjoy it. I normally attend the 90-minute session in the morning before I eat anything, because Bikram recommends that you not eat for 2–3 hours before a session.

After moderate exercise, my glucose reading normally comes down about 30–40 points. With Bikram, it is 20–25 points higher. Why? Is such strenuous exercise safe for me?

Name Withheld

Bret Goodpaster, PhD, responds:

What to Know: Different types of exercise may influence your blood glucose in very different ways. It is well known that both the intensity and duration of the exercise are key reasons for blood glucose levels going either up or down.

There are several possible explanations of why your blood glucose could be elevated with more strenuous, longer-duration exercise such as Bikram yoga. During this more strenuous exercise in the heat, it is likely that your body is producing more of the "stress hormones" such as epinephrine (a.k.a. adrenaline) as well as glucagon, which can certainly raise blood glucose. What's more, heat, humidity, and possible dehydration can act as additional stresses. Elevation in blood glucose with this type of strenuous exercise is a normal hormonal and stress response.

Find Out More: Although a rise of 20–25 points in blood glucose might not be dangerous, it partly depends on your glucose level at the start of exercise. I would advise against this type of strenuous workout if your fasting blood glucose is near 300 mg/dl. If, however, your blood glucose levels are not going into the 300-plus range even after the workout, and your health-care provider has indicated that you are otherwise healthy to exercise, this type of yoga may be OK. The long-term health benefits of intensive exercise may outweigh a small, temporary elevation in blood glucose levels.

Takeaways: Congratulations on getting regular exercise! Although you may enjoy Bikram yoga, there are frankly too many unpredictable variables involved (high intensity, heat, humidity, possible dehydration) for me to be able to say unconditionally that this particular form of exercise is absolutely safe for you.

How Should I Deal with Airport Security?

I wear both an insulin pump and a continuous glucose monitor (CGM), which in the past have set off alarms in airport magnetometers, resulting in pat-down searches. Now, with major airports using the new body imaging equipment for screening passengers, will my devices be harmed by the new scanners? Should I request the more invasive pat-down?

S. L., Indian Head Park, IL

Christy Parkin, MSN, RN, CDE, responds: The American Diabetes Association has been in communication with the Transportation Security Administration (TSA) since its founding in 2001. The Association is part of the TSA's Disability Coalition and works on alerting the TSA staff to problems with security screening procedures.

The TSA's screening procedures for passengers involve full-body scanning and sometimes pat-downs. The body checks are for people who opt out of using the new imaging scanners and traditional metal detectors, and for those who cause an alarm to sound when going through the metal detectors.

Because diabetes presents challenges during airport security screenings (carrying sharp objects, liquids, and devices that TSA agents may not be familiar with), your best defense is to be prepared. It is important to know your rights. You are permitted by law to wear your insulin pump and CGM system through security. Print a copy of the most up-to-date information from the TSA website and take it with you. Allow plenty of time to pass through airport security.

If you go through a scanner and an irregularity is picked up, you should be inspected only at the site of the irregularity (for example, your pump site). If you are concerned about going through a metal detector or scanner with your pump, notify the security officer that you are wearing a pump and would like a full-body pat-down and a visual inspection of your pump instead. Tell the officer that the pump can't be removed because it is attached with a catheter (tubing) under the skin. If a screener tries to remove your pump or CGM system, ask for a supervisor to intervene. You have a right to have somebody with you to witness any additional screening and to have the screening in a private location, if you wish.

Product guidelines for some, but not all, devices suggest that pump-wearers should not go through the scan or send the devices on the conveyor belt through the metal detector. If in doubt before traveling, call your pump and CGM company, and ask for the most recent position statement on your particular device. Obviously, you don't want to damage your expensive electronic equipment by going through a body scanner. The only alternative at this time is a pat-down.

Although some travelers have reported that people with insulin pumps are undergoing an extensive check of all their carry-on bags, not just medical supplies, this is no longer official TSA policy, as a result of the American Diabetes Association's advocacy. For most people with diabetes, going through airport security is completely incident-free, so you shouldn't feel afraid to fly. But if you think that you might encounter a problem, contact TSA Cares (1-855-787-2227), a helpline that assists people with medical conditions and disabilities. You can call 72 hours in advance to request support at the airport.

The American Diabetes Association continues to monitor TSA guidelines, policies, and practices, advocates for change when necessary, and regularly posts updated information at www.diabetes.org/airportsecurity. If you believe you have been subjected to any unfair treatment because of your diabetes, please contact 1-800-DIABETES (1-800-342-2383) and ask to speak with a legal advocate. The advocate can speak with you about the incident and give you information on your rights. The advocate will encourage you to contact the TSA Office for Civil Rights (OCR) as well to report any incident. The OCR is generally able to get to the bottom of problems, often by retraining employees who haven't followed procedures properly or who have failed to treat travelers with the respect they deserve. In some cases, with the individual's permission, the Association will contact TSA directly.

Does Diabetes
Cause Fatigue?

I am a 55-year-old man with type 2 diabetes who is on oral medi-cation. I find that I am very tired in the afternoon. Is this a side effect of diabetes? If so, can anything be done about it?

Name Withheld

Robert A. Gabbay, MD, PhD, responds: A feeling of tiredness and fatigue is often a difficult symptom to try to explain. It can be caused by so many different factors. In people with diabetes, those can include anything from hypothyroidism to heart disease to anemia that is related to kidney disease, to name a few.

Both hypoglycemia (low blood glucose) and hyperglycemia (high blood glucose) can cause fatigue. Checking your blood glucose when you feel tired is an important step, to be sure that it is not too low or too high. If you do have hypoglycemia, then the diabetes medication certainly could be the cause of your tiredness. If there is no hypoglycemia, however, oral medications for diabetes do not typically cause fatigue.

Is Diabetes Caused by Surgery Different?

I had 60% of my pancreas removed because of kidney cancer. I was left with insulin-dependent diabetes. Is surgically induced diabetes treated like other types?

J. A. E., Salisbury, MA

Paris Roach, MD, responds:

What to Know: Diabetes due to pancreatectomy—the surgical removal of the entire pancreas—is similar to type 1 diabetes, in which the immune system destroys the insulin-producing β-cells of the pancreas. Although type 1 diabetes is characterized by complete loss of insulin production, the loss of pancreatic function is more extensive with total pancreatectomy. Not only is insulin absent, but the glucose-balancing hormone glucagon goes away as well, the pancreas being its only source. In addition, digestive enzymes previously produced by the pancreas have to be taken in pill form with meals.

Find Out More: Glucagon's action is opposite that of insulin. It acts to raise blood glucose and in a way "balances" insulin's action of lowering blood glucose. So, you might assume that the treatment of diabetes due to pancreatectomy would be associated with an increased risk of hypoglycemia (low blood glucose) compared with type 1 diabetes, in which glucagon is present, although sometimes at lower levels. However, a Mayo Clinic review of 137 patients followed for an average of 2–3 years after pancreatectomies found that the incidence of hypoglycemia, including severe hypoglycemia (requiring someone else's help to treat), and diabetic ketoacidosis was roughly equal between pancreatectomy and typical type 1 diabetes populations.[2] Mild, self-treated hypoglycemia is not uncommon in either group, but severe hypoglycemia is generally infrequent. Some pancreatectomy patients have nutritional and gastrointestinal issues that may complicate diabetes management.

Most people who undergo partial pancreatectomy do not develop diabetes. Exceptions include people with diseases such as pancreatitis or a family history of diabetes. Because you had a partial pancreatectomy, your body still may produce some insulin. Although it will not be enough insulin to prevent diabetes, it may make your blood glucose levels a bit easier to manage.

Takeaways: Management of both type 1 diabetes and diabetes due to pancreatectomy is a balancing act between too much and too little insulin. Being vigilant in self-management and working with your care team can help you set reasonable glucose targets while minimizing your risk of hypoglycemia.

2 Parsaik AK, Murad MH, Sathananthan A, Moorthy V, Erwin PJ, Chari S, Carter RE, Farnell MB, Vege SS, Sarr MG, Kudva YC. Metabolic and target organ outcomes after total pancreatectomy: Mayo Clinic experience and meta-analysis of the literature. *Clin Endocrinol.* 2010 Dec;73(6):723-731.

Diabetes Forecast®, The Healthy Living Magazine, is the premier lifestyle magazine for people with diabetes, helping you and your family thrive. The magazine shares information backed by the American Diabetes Association and the authentic voices of people living with diabetes. The print, digital, and online issues are all included in your subscription.

Enjoy accurate and timely information about diet, fitness, self-care, and research breakthroughs. Be inspired by the people in our diabetes community. Try something new and delicious every day of the year with our easy recipes. *Diabetes Forecast* is your trustworthy friend for better health!

Subscribe & Save!
Subscribe to *Diabetes Forecast* today at our
SPECIAL ASK THE EXPERTS SAVINGS.

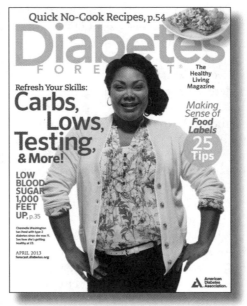

Best Value! 2 years (24 months) of *Diabetes Forecast* for $19—SAVE 84% off the newsstand price—or 1 year (12 months) of *Diabetes Forecast* for $12.

Three Ways to Order Instantly:
1. Call 1-800-806-7801, mention offer code: **M3BATE**
2. Go to www.diabetes.org/askexperts
3. Send your name and address with payment to:
   American Diabetes Association
   Membership Department
   P.O. Box 1643
   Merrifield, VA 22116-9856